AF088352

Dispensing Death and Destruction for Only a Few Pence

Dispensing Death and Destruction for Only a Few Pence

The Nadir of Elizabeth Vamplew, Aged 13

Malcolm Moyes

Copyright © 2024 Malcolm Moyes

The moral right of the author has been asserted.

Apart from any fair dealing for the purposes of research or private study, or criticism or review, as permitted under the Copyright, Designs and Patents Act 1988, this publication may only be reproduced, stored or transmitted, in any form or by any means, with the prior permission in writing of the publishers, or in the case of reprographic reproduction in accordance with the terms of licences issued by the Copyright Licensing Agency. Enquiries concerning reproduction outside those terms should be sent to the publishers.

Troubador Publishing Ltd
Unit E2 Airfield Business Park
Harrison Road, Market Harborough
Leicestershire LE16 7UL
Tel: 0116 279 2299
Email: books@troubador.co.uk
Web: www.troubador.co.uk

ISBN 978-1-80514-281-2

British Library Cataloguing in Publication Data.
A catalogue record for this book is available from the British Library.

Printed and bound by CPI Group (UK) Ltd, Croydon, CR0 4YY
Typeset in 12pt Minion Pro by Troubador Publishing Ltd, Leicester, UK

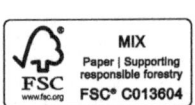

'Some may think it odd for a man to sit down and write on so trifling a subject as Vermin'

The Complete Vermin killer or Gentleman's and Farmer's Guide for Destroying Water-Rats, House Rats, Field Rats, Mice, Moles, Ants, or Pissmires, Worms, Snails, Grasshoppers, Crows, Weazels, Polecats, Stoats and Foxes, in a Plain and Easy Manner, Compiled after Twenty Years' Experience by Thomas Simpson, Grazier, in the East Riding of Yorkshire (published by John Smith, York, 1772)

Contents

Acknowledgements ix
Introduction xi

Chapter One
Prologue to murder, suicide and self-harm:
a short history of vermin killers 1

Chapter Two
'A person exceedingly dangerous': a short
history of Elizabeth Vamplew, aged thirteen
years 109
Bibliography 178

Acknowledgements

I would like to thank the British Library which, through its digital archives of C19th and C20th newspapers, enabled me to access with relative ease the news reports, adverts and articles relating to eighteenth and nineteenth century vermin killers, as well as to the trial of Elizabeth Vamplew.

I am also indebted to the National Archives at Kew, which supplied me with copies of the Home Office documents relating to the trial, imprisonment and subsequent release of Elizabeth Vamplew.

The Wellcome Institute in London, through its on-line library, enabled me to consult various rare early books on the subject of vermin killing, and gave kind permission to reproduce the *Hunter's Infallible Vermin and Insect Killer* label from its collection.

My thanks are also due to the staff of Sleaford and Lincoln libraries for their invaluable support in providing access to material in their local history collections, as well as obtaining scarce out of print books through the inter-library loan system.

I would like to thank, once again, the staff of the Lincolnshire Archives for their unfailing help and courtesy in giving me access to the various documents in their collections.

Finally, I would like to express my gratitude to Paul and Emma at Good Finds Antiques in Heckington, for allowing me to reproduce the excerpt taken from a C19th chemist's book of commercial preparations.

Introduction

In his book, *Victorian Things,* the distinguished historian, Asa Briggs, constructed an understanding of the nineteenth century by analysing the significance of the ordinary and the everyday.

His terms of reference for the concept of the ordinary and everyday were numerous and wide ranging:

'I wanted to consider the *things* which they designed, named, made, advertised, bought and sold, listed, counted, collected, gave to others, threw away or bequeathed.'

More broadly, and borrowing an idea originally found in T S Eliot's *Notes Towards the Definition of a Culture*, he wished to explore the object in question as 'an emissary of the culture out of which it comes'.

As a caveat to his proposed ambitious sweep of Victorian society, Professor Briggs admitted that his selection of things left much out, and further, that because most people were poor they had little or no access to the things which he analysed and reflected upon in the course of his book.

One such emissary of commercial culture not included in the book, to which the poor certainly did have access, was vermin killer, a thing which answers to most of the descriptors found in the check list offered by Professor Briggs, with the exceptions, unsurprisingly, of it being collected or bequeathed in a will. Nineteenth century vermin killers were designed for a specific purpose to meet a specific need; packaged and identified by name; produced by a variety of people throughout the century and beyond; widely advertised in newspapers; bought and sold in small villages and large cities; listed amongst such everyday essentials as *Singleton's Eye-Cream* and *Godfrey's Cordial*; given to others, including many who would rather not have had it; and was occasionally thrown away, often as a quick and easy solution to the uncomfortable truth of having owned it in the first place.

Hardly a thing of beauty, its qualities of public and private utility were undeniable: it was cheap, efficient and did what it said on the packet, with impressive results: it dispensed sudden death to the undesirable.

The suggestion that vermin killer has a strong case for inclusion in any list of Victorian things which were emissaries of the culture that produced it, is further strengthened by noting just a few of the key messages which it despatched, both overtly and covertly, to the customer.

Vermin killer had serious military connotations, amounting to a declaration of war, being sold as an effective weapon against an enemy which was both rapacious and devious. Rats and mice in particular were notorious criminals of the natural world, living freely without scruples concerning the destruction and misery which they caused in the house and on the farms of respectable people. They were a universal social problem in need of an efficient universal cure, based upon superior human ingenuity and efficiency, as well as being a cheap, progressive improvement on the past.

More importantly, vermin killers made serious money for the men who manufactured them on an industrial scale, for the men who sold them in their shops and, at the same time, saved money for the men and women who bought them to combat the common enemy. There was also the added commercial advantage, neither advertised nor admitted, that as long as social conditions in general remained insanitary and houses, both rural and urban, remained squalid, there would always be a pressing need to buy the product. As long as the problem persisted, nineteenth century householders, farmers, warehouse owners and ship's captains would remain consumers of the various brands of vermin killer on the market.

Whilst destructive economic forces, unbridled human greed, ineffectual legislation, inequality between men and woman, predatory abusive behaviours and the studied complacency of the rich and powerful continued to exist, vulnerable people would also remain consumers, in turn themselves becoming consumed in the many appalling newspaper stories of self-harm, suicide and murder.

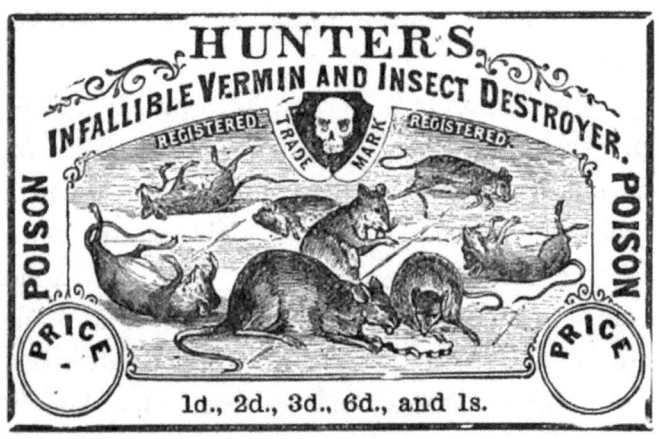

Chapter One

Prologue to murder, suicide and self-harm: a short history of vermin killers

Before the mass production and distribution of commercial vermin killers in the nineteenth century, there were various small-scale solutions available to deal with any unwanted incursions of wildlife, some more effective than others. On the one hand, there was a diverse range of traditional approaches, passed on from generation to generation, some of which became fixed in handy manuals instructing the concerned reader on how to set about dealing with the perennial problem of vermin. On the other hand, there was always recourse to the local apothecary who dispensed his own particular concoctions which, in all probability, were just a recycling of familiar traditional solutions with an added twist.

Whilst it is clear that rats and mice were the most problematic and persistent of the uninvited guests which plagued daily life, the hit-lists of common vermin in urgent need of elimination found in books and unpublished manuscripts, were remarkably comprehensive.

To some extent, this is attributable to the context of such hints and advice on the management of vermin being part of more general accounts of agricultural good practice, aimed primarily at an audience of gentlemen farmers: it was unlikely that any town-dweller would have had any serious issues with adders, badgers or otters.

Pre-nineteenth century solutions to the problem of destroying vermin were a predictable mix of the obvious, the ridiculous and the downright dangerous. In most cases, they were also inefficient and labour intensive, requiring a breezy optimism that the behaviour of rats and mice, in particular, was entirely predictable, and that after a few nights of taking heavy casualties they would soon decamp and go somewhere else.

One of the most remarkable books offering advice on the effective destruction of rats and mice was published and sold by a consortium of booksellers in London, around 1725. The linguistically mangled title promised useful hints on the care of cattle and the maintenance of gardens, but mainly comprehensive advice on vermin control:

> *The compleat English, French, and High-German Vermin-killer. To which is added, directions for curing all sorts of cattle. With some directions for gardiners: being a Companion for all Families shewing A ready way to destroy Adders, Badgers, Birds of all sorts, Bugs, Ducks, Earwigs, Fish, Fleas, flies, Foxes, Frogs, Gnats, Lice, Mice, Otters, Pismires, Polt-Cats, Rabits, Rats, Scorpions, Snakes, Snails, Spiders, Toads, Wahts or Miles, Wasps, Weasles, Wolf-fly, Worms in Houses, Gardens et cetera, to which is added Directions for Curing all Sorts of Cattle, With some Directions for Gardiners and the Prozes of Workmen's Labour. Being a Rich Cabinet of Curiosities.*

The anonymous book was essentially an expanded new edition of a similarly titled book published earlier on in the century, also in London, by Mr G Conyers at the Ring, located in Little Britain. A good deal of its content was either silently reproduced or slightly modified by many other publications over the next hundred years.

A perusal of the sections of the book dealing with the destruction of rats and mice especially gives the impression that the professed intention of the author to offer the last word on the subject was an earnest one. Drawing upon classical authors such as Pliny the Elder, and more modern authorities, such as the German occultist Heinrich Cornelius Agrippa, plus a wide range of folk lore culled from earlier English writers, the compiler provided many reassurances and guarantees, most of them highly questionable.

The use of cats and traps was acknowledged as the common and effective way of dealing with rats and mice, although the claim that they might account for a hundred victims in one night seemed more than a little fanciful, even in Hamelin.

Most of the advice related to the judicious and injudicious use of herbs, sugar and poisons in various combinations, which were to be mixed into a paste before being strategically placed.

The use of a mixture of a pennyworth of treacle with bird-lime, for example, was precisely described as requiring the sticky pellets to be 'as big as a hazel nut' and to be placed on a piece of paper 'the breadth of a shilling', so that the unsuspecting vermin trod in it and tried to lick the substance off its feet. With undisguised triumph, the writer noted, without the least hint of any distracting sentimentality, that the consumption of the paste 'burns their guts'.

Yet more brutal was the mixing of powdered ratsbane with butter, barley and honey, which was to be left on trenchers or boards: the arsenic generated a raging thirst and the creature would drink 'until it bursts'. Given the power of the poison, the writer very responsibly warned the readers to wash their hands after preparing such a dangerous mixture.

A more sophisticated solution to the problem of rodent infestation involved a preparation of quicksilver, black hellebore and the seed of wild cucumber, to be added to a small piece of meat: quite simply, the culprits ate it and they died. It was a preparation, the writer advised, which was readily available from an apothecary or druggist.

If the end product of vermin killer was a painful death, the process of some of the remedies for ridding a house of the problem in one go amounted to calculated cruelty. With the precision of a cookery book, the reader was instructed to 'take a rat or mouse and beat him, or cut him sore', so that once he had been let go, 'he'll cry and make such a noise that it will fright all the rest of the house'. Even more grotesque was the anecdotal information that some people 'take them and fleece the skin off their heads', which produced a similar fearful exodus from the house. It is not surprising that at least one later writer on the subject thought this method too cruel to even contemplate.

Some of the more outlandish instructions to the reader involved the unsavoury use of the body parts of dead animals to drive vermin away from any room which might contain food, especially cheese.

Citing the authority of Agrippa on the matter, the reader is instructed to mix hog's lard with the brains of a weasel, which when made into pellets and left in a room, would deter any rat or mouse from entering. Any doubt about the usefulness of the remedy, or concern about its possible impact on the comfort of any guests, was countered by the writer's one word definitive judgement: 'Approved'.

The usefulness of the weasel as a vermin deterrent seems to have had a venerable history, as the writer cites Pliny's observation that the ashes of a weasel would also do the job, as would the ashes of a cat dropped into water and then sprinkled around the house. Unfortunately, the writer was unable to offer his usual reassuring seal of approval to either of these dubious suggestions.

Less repugnant solutions, many of which were approved by the writer, involved burning various plants, such as wild celery, wild marjoram, nigella, lupin and tamarind, or merely scenting the room with bog-myrtle, traditionally used as an insect repellent.

Thomas Simpson, an East Yorkshire grazier, in his practical manual of vermin killing published in 1772, was in no doubt that rats should be seen not as a tricky domestic problem, but more as an alarming national plague:

> '...we are clearly convinced, to our sorrow, that every part of the Isle is pestered by them; this Rat will not only frequent barns, but ricks, sewers, hen-houses, hog-sties, under floors, in houses, behind wainscots, and ceilings.'

He also noted that the nobility and farmers were in the habit of employing rat-catchers to sort out the problem, but Thomas Simpson clearly had serious reservations on the matter. The rat-catcher's fee was based upon the number of rats which he caught in his trap that night: regrettably, some unscrupulous members of the rat-catching fraternity were in the habit of recycling the catch 'half a dozen times' with a consequent increase in employer expenditure without any happy decrease in the rat population. The common sense solution, other than not employing a rat-catcher at all, was to insist that each rat presented, supposedly caught, but probably purchased for the occasion, had its head cut off on the spot.

According to Thomas Simpson, there was a further limitation to employing a rat-catcher beyond the question of trust and honesty, which was based upon the efficacy of his methods.

One favoured method of removing rats from

barns and houses, for example, was to stab them with a 'long spear' which sometimes hit the target, but more often than not just made holes in the thatching through which the rain could seep.

The ubiquitous steel and wooden traps, baited with only cheese and bacon, were not entirely reliable either: what was required was a more sophisticated preparation, involving the careful mixing into a paste of three large spoonfuls of flour, three spoonfuls of grated white bread, one spoonful of treacle, three drops of caraway oil, three drops of aniseed oil and six drops of a red herring oil. After the trap was set with the bait, it would then be necessary to scent it with half an ounce of oil of rhodium, half an ounce of oil of caraway, half an ounce of oil of aniseed and finally, with two grains of musk.

The precision of Thomas Simpson's instructions was only matched by a worthy anxiety about the safety of people. Repeating concerns found in earlier books, he noted that contraptions left out in an open field represented a possible danger to the unaware; he therefore recommended that when a field had been cleared, a bait of hemlock seeds with either flour or honey, mixed with ox-vomit and mashed into a paste should be placed at the entrance of the hole used by the rats. In a state of some excitement at the thought of making a significant contribution to solving the national rat crisis, Mr Simpson claimed that the bait would 'immediately destroy all rats in the field'.

In his characterisation of mice, Thomas Simpson, was perhaps even more plain-speaking than in his description of rats: the house mouse had 'a very devouring and nasty nature', whilst his cousin, the field mouse, was 'very pernicious'. The same vermin killer used for rats, consisting of finely powdered hemlock seeds, flour or honey and ox-vomit, was prescribed, also promising to 'destroy all that feed upon it'.

Whether it was a question of trusting proven traditional methods for killing vermin, a personal dislike of rat-catchers or a requirement to bulk out a book, Thomas Simpson presented a range of alternative 'receipts' for killing rats and mice, as well as other pests, many of which he had copied from earlier eighteenth-century books on the subject.

But such men as Thomas Simpson had virtually had their day, their advice and instructions surviving in later household commonplace books and memoranda as ephemeral transcriptions or imperfectly remembered fragments, alongside remedies for such common ailments as rheumatism and coughs. By the early nineteenth century, vermin killer manuals, with their staple offering of deadly poison, ancient recipes and nonsense, were in decline. Whilst such relics of the late eighteenth, such as Daniel

Holland's *Universal Vermin Killer* persisted and existed on the library shelves of the nobility and well-to-do farmers, they were being superseded by robust commercial enterprise which not only provided a ready-made deadly product in a convenient packet, but also a set of handy instructions for its application both in the home and on the farm.

In the last decade of the eighteenth century, the lucrative commercial possibilities of the sale of solutions to the rat problem were recognised by Thomas Reiss, a Hampshire grain merchant, who claimed to have invented an infallible vermin killer. Sold in a distinctive packet sealed with an impressed red stamp of the Havant Mill, near Portsmouth, and marketed as *The Hampshire Miller's Rat Powder*, the product was originally sold in London, but became more widely available 'at all reputable booksellers and stationers in the country'. Judging by the disgruntled notices appearing from time to time in various provincial newspapers in the 1790s, which complained about the shameless trade in counterfeits of his product, the vermin killer was a commercial success. Despite such outrageous sharp practices involving 'spurious compositions' *The Hampshire Miller's Infallible Rat Powder* was still being successfully sold, at least in the shop of Knight & Son in Windsor, in 1814.

By the middle of the nineteenth century, if you

weren't a big fan of mice, rats and beetles, serious help was increasingly on hand: whether it was an annoying intrusion into domestic pantries and cellars or a challenging infestation of agricultural produce stored in the barn, various commercial products were becoming widely available, which were both cheap and effective.

Products on the market to sort out personal and professional aversions to such noxious creatures were numerous and all of them, of course, promised instant results for the beleaguered householder or farmer faced with the problem of vermin.

In 1846, *Butler's Vermin Killer*, known also as *Butler's Vermin and Insect Killer*, as well as *Butler's Gloucestershire Vermin and Insect Killer*, seemed to establish an early market dominance, with a savvy marketing strategy of advertising well beyond the charming Cotswold town of Wooton under Edge, where the product originated. According to William Butler, his solution not only offered complete reassurance to farmers and housekeepers that any unwelcome guests would be instantly killed, but also to mill owners, ship masters, inn keepers and even 'professed vermin destroyers'.

The sale of over three hundred thousand packets of *Butler's Vermin Killer* by May, 1846, was encouraging, but so were the frequent testimonials liberally stuffed with plain-speaking hyperbole, which accompanied the regular newspaper adverts promoting the product. Mr Simco of Northampton, clearly having endured a distressing long-term problem with beetles, celebrated the fact that after using *Butler's Vermin Killer* he awoke the next morning to discover 'the black-coated detestables all dead'. R H Minchin, Commander of the brig, *Maria*, described his ship as 'swarming with mice and rats', but after the application of a shilling packet of *Butler's Vermin Killer*, much to his astonishment, even the furry variety of detestables had 'entirely disappeared'.

Adverts for *Butler's Vermin Killer* not only drew attention to the testimonials of delighted customers, but also to endorsements from highly satisfied shop keepers who were clearly making decent profits from stocking the product. Mr W D Allot of Sheffield stated that he had 'sold a considerable quantity', and had 'just ordered a further supply'; whilst Mr John Walker of Bradford voiced his approval by confirming that he had sold *Butler's Vermin Killer* for three years and found that 'the demand increases every day'.

Perhaps in an attempt to persuade the reader that the packet of deadly poison was as much a social service as it was a commercial enterprise, the adverts also cited the admiring approval of popular newspapers and magazines. The *Sheffield Iris*, for example, was of the opinion that Mr Butler had 'laid all classes under deep obligation', whilst according to the *Blackwood's Ladies Magazine*, the publication was doing its readers a great kindness, as well as performing a public duty, by drawing attention to Mr Butler's preparation.

In addition to ensuring death and destruction to some of the less attractive inhabitants of the natural world, William Butler was also anxious to make it clear to all concerned purchasers that any accident from its use was 'next to impossible', on account of its dark colour and having an offensive odour. Further, and assuming that his patrons were literate, all packets of poison were accompanied by a clear set of directions to aid its ease of application.

Butler's Vermin Killer was indisputably a commercial success and was still being stocked in chemist's shops in the late 1880s.

Hot on the heels of commercial success, unashamed imitation inevitably follows: within a short space of time, Mr John Richard Battle of Lincoln, announced to the world the availability of *Battle's Vermin Killer*. Building on the good fortune of the similar sounding name of the two products, Battle also spent copious amounts of money on advertising the brutal efficacy of his product, accompanied by the testimonials of purchasers who, happily, were now no longer plagued by rats, mice and other assorted nuisances.

People who bought *Battle's Vermin Killer* were as delighted with the merchandise as were the purchasers of *Butler's Vermin Killer*, it seems. In an advert placed in *Bell's Weekly Messenger*, 20th December, 1852, just two years after its introduction, it was claimed that over eighty thousand packets of the product had been sold that year and that enthusiastic testimonials ran into their thousands. The often repeated suggestion from one of its purchasers that *Battle's Vermin Killer* was 'getting into great fame' seemed an understatement, if the claims of such rapid large scale commercial success were true.

William Butler and John Richard Battle had identified a lucrative opportunity in the market and had responded to it with admirable entrepreneurial energy. In turn, their success encouraged other commercial enterprises to also try and grab a share of any opportunities available to make good money from fear and loathing.

Hunter's Vermin Killer, later rebranded as *Hunter's Infallible Vermin and Insect Destroyer*, enjoyed a good deal of commercial success between the early 1850s and the 1880s: like *Battle's Vermin Killer*, it contained strychnine, and was sometimes marketed alongside it by chemists and druggists as the most effective low-cost antidote available to the ills inflicted on society by rats and mice.

Mr Harper Twelvetrees, an East London entrepreneur and philanthropist, formerly a grocer located on Church Street, Boston, and well-known for his glycerine soap powders, was a surprising late entrant into the market. With his customary ebullience and determination, the author of *The Science of Washing* implemented a national newspaper campaign to promote *Twelvetrees's Mice and Rat Killer* in the late 1850s, blitzing the entire of the United Kingdom with his playful commercial irony: 'the most delicious dainty ever prepared for vermin', he observed of his latest product, which was now widely available to ensure that mice and rats dropped down dead on the spot.

Unsurprisingly, smaller, less ambitious products also appeared on the market, which adopted a similar promotional approach by way of newspaper columns, whilst sometimes trying to make their commercial offer distinctive from that of the bigger players.

In Lincolnshire, numerous resourceful chemists and druggists both produced and marketed their own preparations, which were sold mainly to a local clientele, especially farmers concerned about the infestation of their haystacks.

The Spalding Chemical Vermin Killer, prepared by Francis Milns, chemist and druggist, located in the Market Place of the town, was promoted as 'the best that has hitherto been introduced for the destruction of rats and mice'. The accompanying list of outlets was impressive, amounting to an assortment of over twenty chemists, booksellers and druggists, scattered around the county. The distinctive attribute of the preparation was that it was 'free from smell and taste' – a feature which provided useful advantages in the war against rats and mice, who 'greedily devour it'; unfortunately, it may have also have provided some fatal disadvantages for domestic pets.

On a less ambitious scale, Samuel Fisher Brett, located on Queen Street, Market Rasen, advertised his own brand of vermin killer in the town, and slightly further afield in Nottingham; whilst John Hewson of Mercer Row, Louth and John Holliday Thomas of Market Place, Boston, plainly and modestly alerted local patrons to the availability of their respective preparations in the unending struggle against vermin in the county. By way of a contrast, George Patterson, an agricultural chemist located in Lion Square, Stamford, (who, incidentally, gave decisive evidence in the sensational matricide trial of the poisoner, Thomas Fuller Bacon), was less restrained in his approach to marketing, boldly advertising his preparation with the striking moniker, *Patterson's Magic Vermin Killer*, well beyond Lincolnshire.

The trend for using this evocative adjective to describe the wondrous destructive powers of poison may well have had its origins in early adverts for *Battle's Vermin Killer*, which claimed that mice 'appear attracted to it as by magic'. The concept was certainly employed to advertise a number of products, some relatively short-lived, whose effectiveness was claimed to be magical rather than chemical, such as *Bartle's Magic Vermin Killer* (Banbury), *Cowan's Magic Vermin Destroyer* (London) and *Emery's Magic Beetle Poison (London)*.

That the vermin killer market became an increasingly competitive one is suggested by the number of warnings embedded in newspaper adverts alerting any naïve readers to the existence of fraudulent, and even dangerous copy-cat products. In 1860, the proprietors of *Hunter's Infallible Vermin Killer*, for example, strongly advised its customers, to beware duplicitous imitations, whilst an outraged John Richard Battle, five years earlier, had expressed alarm that some unscrupulous parties were 'endeavouring to push the sale of a vile imitation'. As late as 1887, the Lincoln chemist's sensitivity to lost revenue compelled him to take out an advert in *The Times*, announcing that he had directed the Trade Mark Protection Society to instruct its solicitors to take legal action against 'any manufacturers, factors or dealers infringing his Registered Labels'.

The ready availability of such remedies may have made a contribution to public health and private profit, but their unfortunate by-product was the death of human beings, sometimes accidentally, sometimes deliberately.

Between 1860 and 1870, *Hunter's Infallible Vermin*

Killer was reported to have been used in one case of infanticide, at least four suicide attempts, one of which was successful, and most involving impoverished or deserted young women. All were distressing, but the murder of five-month old Edward John Thompson, the illegitimate son of unemployed bridle stitcher, Lucy Thompson, in Birmingham, in 1868, was particularly so. The twenty-year old had been turned out her lodgings and the father of the child had taken no interest in her destitute state, leaving her to wander the streets, hungry and penniless, before finally spending the night in a graveyard, where she administered *Hunter's Infallible Vermin Killer* to her son. Described by the newspaper reports of the time as 'a wretched looking object' and 'always of weak intellect', she was found Not Guilty of wilful murder on the grounds of insanity at the Warwick Assizes, but was detained indefinitely at Her Majesty's displeasure, alongside other inconvenient casualties of an unequal society.

The story of eighteen-year old Elizabeth Kent of Netherton, Gloucestershire, in 1866, who attempted to commit suicide after hearing local gossip which suggested that she was pregnant, was an instructive one in terms of the gloomy history of the easy availability of vermin killer laced with strychnine. Clearly in a state of some distress after being cruelly discarded by the putative father, she had bought a packet of *Hunter's Infallible Vermin Killer* from Mr Arkell, the local chemist, on the familiar pretence of having a problem with mice. Interestingly, she had at first asked Thomas Powell, the assistant to Mr Arkell, to sell her a packet of *Battle's Vermin Killer*, but she did not have enough money; instead, and without question, she was offered a packet of *Hunter's Infallible Vermin Killer*, as a cheaper solution to her pressing problem: Mr Arkell was clearly well stocked and on-trend.

Whilst packets of vermin killer in general were probably responsible for as many unrecorded deaths as recorded ones in the second half of the nineteenth-century, it was *Battle's Vermin Killer* which appears to have been the product of choice for anyone wishing to end their life, or that of others. An early testimonial published in the *Stamford Mercury,* 1st February, 1850, provided not only an enthusiastic endorsement of the product, but also an unintended grim forecast of its misuse, as the century progressed: 'Your killer is a killer indeed, and make no mistake'.

The number of recorded cases of suicide or attempted suicide involving *Battle's Vermin Killer* in Lincolnshire alone appears to have surpassed that of all other similar products combined.

Inevitably, there were a large number of cases of young women, caught up in a seemingly hopeless situation, where there seemed to be no alternative other than to seek salvation in a threepenny packet of strychnine.

In September, 1862, the case of Ann Tilson, in the service of a Mrs Duckett of the Ship Inn, Bardney, was brought before the magistrates. Unsympathetically described by the *Lincolnshire Chronicle* as 'a foolish girl', she had attempted to end her life with a packet of *Battle's Vermin Killer*, seemingly as a result of personal difficulties with a young man, 'who had been paying his addresses to her'. Fortunately, Ann Tillson received medical treatment in time to save her life and her mother, in her daughter's absence from court, was able to give re-assurances that she would not attempt to end her life again.

There was no such outcome for eighteen-year old Mary Hodson who, the following month, poisoned herself in the borough gaol, after appearing in front of the Grantham magistrates on the charge of stealing a quantity of clothing from the house and shop of her master, Thomas Wand.

The two accounts of the inquest into her death, published in the *Grantham Journal* and the *Lincolnshire Chronicle*, suggest a degree of awkwardness about the circumstances of the case. In addition to the young woman having managed to poison herself whilst incarcerated in a gaol and therefore under guard, it was clear that the coroner, Mr W G Wagstaffe, was uneasy that the five local doctors involved in looking into the case could not agree upon a precise and definitive cause of death, even after chemical analysis.

These issues were to some extent resolved, at least to the apparent satisfaction of the coroner, through a deft mix of judicious direction and tactful reminders to the jury of the potential cost of justice to the public purse.

It seemed clear that Mary Hodson had died as a result of strychnine poisoning, but the finer points of the case relating to how and where she had acquired the deadly substance appeared to be left conveniently unresolved. In terms of a secure analysis of the stomach and viscera of the young girl, the jury was invited to make a judgement based purely on the conflicting evidence of the Grantham medical men, as the cost of at least £50 to procure the expert services of Professor Swaine Taylor of Guy's Hospital was deemed prohibitive.

The final verdict of the jury, although not all of the jury, was that Mary Hodson had died from the effects of poison administered by her own hand, in a fit of temporary insanity, rather than *felo de se*. The speculative final verdict of the *Lincolnshire Chronicle*, based upon remarks made by just one of the Grantham doctors, was that Mary Hodson had ended her life quite deliberately with a quantity of *Battle's Vermin Killer,* which she had possibly stolen from the house of her employer, Mr Wand.

The easy verdict that young women who chose to end their lives in such a dreadful way was due to insanity, temporary or otherwise, to some extent, became a means of avoiding difficult conversations with clerics and insurance companies.

Such judgements also helped to explain away the annoyingly inexplicable. The actions of hapless, lovestruck servant girls were obviously caused by fatal attractions of a most unfortunate kind, but those of apparently respectable married women intent on destroying themselves with vermin killer, was less comfortable material for public consumption.

The suicide of twenty-six year old Mary Ann Knight, the wife of Sleaford shoemaker, Edward Knight, and the subsequent inquest at the Bristol Arms in the town, was reported twice by the *Lincolnshire Chronicle*, but in versions so divergent that the reader may well have been left in a state of total confusion as to what really happened.

The earliest report of 12th December, 1862, made it clear that the actions of Mrs Knight had been meticulously planned. She had called at the shop of Charles Petchell, the local druggist, asking for poison to deal with an infestation of mice. He had offered her *Battle's Vermin Killer*, as an obvious solution, but she chose instead to purchase a stronger alternative, prepared by the chemist himself. After securing the poison, she then visited the shop of the confectioner, Mr William Elmore, from whom Mrs Knight bought jam in which to mix an unidentified powder. On reaching home, she retired to bed with her husband and she died during the course of the night.

The post mortem revealed 'strychnine in a large proportion', leading to a verdict of temporary insanity by the coroner's jury. The brisk, matter of fact report seemed oddly short on detail, with few serious questions being asked of the chemist relating to the dispensing of the poison or of the husband concerning the care of his wife in her dying hours.

The second report of the same inquest, published on the 19th December, provided a good deal more detail, but in so doing created a narrative totally at odds with the earlier account: instead of a puzzling suicide by a respectable married woman, the story of Mary Ann Knight was turned into a half-realised, sleazy story of adultery with a young man, whose identity remained predictably elusive. A flat factual story of domestic misfortune only seven days later was transformed into a sensationalist narrative which diverted attention away from awkward questions of commercial propriety and domestic responsibility.

Mary Ann Knight had certainly obtained vermin killer from Charles Petchell, but according to the later of the two reports, she had been served by William Brewin, an assistant to the druggist, who had sold her two pennyworth of rat poison, which consisted of strychnine, lard and cinnabar contained in a pill box.

Thomas Jacobson, surgeon of Sleaford, revealed that he had discovered raspberry jam, a greasy compound and strychnine in the stomach of Mrs Knight, whilst Police Superintendent Edward Pearman confirmed that he had found a pink pill box suspiciously 'stuffed behind some things in a cupboard'. The surgeon also stated that Mary Ann Knight was three months pregnant when she committed suicide, and offered his professional opinion that 'women in that state are liable to become depressed and of a morbid state of mind, with strange fancies'. For this reason, such women may not be accountable for their actions, he suggested.

In contrast to the simple scientific opinion provided by the medical man, a murky picture emerged of Mrs Knight having formed an illicit relationship with a young man in the town with whom she was intending to elope. Such revelations were news to Edward Knight, it seems, as he had believed that he lived on good terms with his wife, although he did concede that her behaviour on the night of her suicide had been unusual and that she had once taken laudanum before they were married 'out of jealousy'.

The jury agreed that Mary Ann Knight had taken strychnine 'in a state of unsound mind', but offered no comment on the precise cause of such extreme unsoundness.

In 1864, the name of Mary Cooke of Gosberton, the wife of a well-established and 'highly respectable' farmer, was added to the dismal litany of Lincolnshire women for whom *Battle's Vermin Killer* had offered a grim exit from existence.

The poor woman, who had previously 'showed signs of aberration of intellect', had been discovered face down in a field, with a bottle of laudanum and numerous fragments of white paper by her side.

On the day that she went missing, Mary Cooke had gone into the shop of Sutterton druggist, William Peach, and had specifically asked for a packet of *Battle's Vermin Killer*. In this she was unsuccessful as Mr Peach said that he had sold out, but luckily he was able to supply her with his own preparation 'which was equally efficacious', as it contained strychnine. In his deposition to the coroner's court at the Swan Inn, Sutterton, William Peach was also keen to explain that the fragments of paper found next to the body of Mary Cooke were definitely part of the wrapper he had used for his own vermin preparation, pointing out a mark where he had gummed the label himself. With equal professional pride, he also drew attention to a small portion of the blue colour of the poison still adhering to wrapper to confirm his evidence. It may have been only a coincidence, but *Battle's Vermin Killer* also contained blue colouring and was a constituent often used as confirmatory evidence by analysts of the agency of the deadly product.

William Peach was keen to also inform the coroner that he did not know Mrs Cooke and that there was 'nothing remarkable in her manner', which might have aroused his suspicion: as with many depositions from druggist and chemists of the time, there was a strong sense of special pleading on the part of Mr Peach, an urgent need to absolve himself from any unsavoury suspicion of carelessness and irresponsibility in the sale of vermin killer in his shop, which might damage business.

The apparent ease with which a determined individual could buy dangerous poisons used for killing vermin, such as nux vomica, was not just down to customer duplicity, however. Professor Alfred Swaine Taylor, the go-to national expert on difficult criminal poison cases, was clearly concerned about a shocking laxity in the sale of such dangerous products.

In a seminal paper published in *The Pharmaceutical Journal and Transactions* (July 1864-June 1865), he expressed unease about the continued lax sale of arsenic despite the existence of the 1851 *Arsenic Act*, describing the law as a 'dead letter'. His criticism, in part, was aimed at chemists and druggists who still sold white arsenic 'on the most frivolous pretences' and thereby 'set the law at defiance'. However, it is clear that his most serious concerns related to uneducated grocers, chandlers, oilmen and village shopkeepers, whose trade in vermin killers and poisons in general, was both unregulated and irresponsible.

In particular, Swaine Taylor was alarmed at the ease with which strychnia and cyanide could be bought 'even by small children' from either the village shop or the local druggist. In this context, he pointed to the easy availability of both *Butler's Vermin Killer* and *Battle's Vermin Killer*, allegedly sold to destroy vermin, but responsible for many cases of suicide and murder, some of which he had first-hand knowledge. A particularly shocking case, in Lincolnshire, involved the murder of an infant by a thirteen-year old girl, who had purchased a three-penny packet of *Battle's Vermin Killer* from the village grocer. Elizabeth Vamplew had procured the product 'without any difficulty' and had put a small portion of the powder into the mouth of an infant, with deadly consequences. Worse still, it was likely that another two infants had died in the same way whilst being cared for by the young girl, who was later tried at the Lincoln Summer Assizes, in 1862, found guilty of manslaughter, and sentenced to penal servitude for twelve years.

Respectable druggists, Professor Taylor conceded, refused to sell such powders, but while ever they were 'a profitable branch of trade in the shops of oilmen, grocers and others', they would remain a serious danger to public health – a danger increased by the fact they were often sold over the counter by naïve and ignorant apprentices.

His gloomy conclusion was that the current situation of cheap and easy access to such products as *Battle's Vermin Killer* was a 'great and unnecessary facility given for destroying human life, under the pretence that the poison was intended for the destruction of vermin'.

His words proved to be horribly prophetic when two young Lincolnshire women, both domestic servants, used *Battle's Vermin Killer* to murder their infant child. Lucy Ann Buxton of Metheringham, near Lincoln, was tried and found guilty of murder, in May 1868, whilst Emma Wade, from Stamford, was similarly tried and convicted in April, 1879. Both women were reprieved by the Home Secretary from the death sentence: Emma Wade, the daughter of a policeman, who attempted suicide as well as committing infanticide, served one year in Lincoln prison; Lucy Ann Buxton, a convicted petty criminal and daughter of a beer house owner, died in Woking prison, Surrey, sometime between 1871 and 1881, her passing marked by a curt, undated marginal note in a prison register.

As well as underlining the urgency of addressing the situation, Taylor's paper also included a lucid ten point action plan which made a significant contribution to improved regulation of the sale of poisons enshrined in the *Pharmacy Act* of 1868.

However, despite a tightening of the law, cases of the misuse of *Battle's Vermin Killer* continued in the rural Lincolnshire throughout the nineteenth century, with appalling regularity, as did the sloppy malpractices of town and village shopkeepers who sold it, despite their self-righteous protestations to the contrary.

Pathetic cases of the misadventures of vulnerable young women continued to fill newspaper columns with their familiar themes of romantic disappointment and oppressive social stigma, as did the harsh judicial outcomes which attributed blame to feckless or temporarily insane individuals, rather than address the blatant societal inadequacies which often generated such misery.

On the 10th July, 1882, twenty-three year old Mary Harvey, from Welbourn, was luckily saved from certain death in Grantham by a passing soldier from the 4th Battalion of the Lincolnshire Regiment, who discovered her sitting on a heap of stones in a Grantham street, and had immediately alerted the police. She had visited two different chemists that morning, buying laudanum, a box of stomach pills and white precipitate at the first shop, and a packet of *Battle's Vermin Killer*, at the second, after having signed the *Poison Register*. The chemist's assistant, William Henry Davies, made it clear to the magistrate that he had no reason to believe that Mary Harvey intended to use it for an illegal purpose: it was a self-evident comment, but clearly one worth making to allay any suspicions of negligence.

That the root of the troubles of Mary Harvey was the recurring one of being abandoned with a child by an errant father was made clear in a lengthy suicide letter addressed to her parents, which was found on her person at the police station. It expressed regret at what she intended to do and pathetically sent 'a kiss for the dear little boy that I love'; it also hoped that her mother would not 'forget to go to the one that had caused my trouble'.

After having consumed both laudanum and *Battle's Vermin Killer*, Mary Harvey was saved by the local surgeon, swiftly despatched to the Union Workhouse to recover and then remanded in custody. Her journey through the legal system continued at the Grantham Quarter Session the following November, but *in absentia*, as she had been committed to the Bracebridge Lunatic Asylum, near Lincoln, on the 21st August, 'by order of the Home Secretary'.

In June, 1883, sixteen-year old Mildred Pepper, the daughter of a Lincoln bricklayer, committed suicide using a packet of *Battle's Vermin Killer*, after becoming involved in an ill-judged relationship with a soldier of the 10th Regiment, aided and abetted by a shady lady by the name of Mrs Brewster. Her father had tried to discourage and then terminate the liaison, and had ended up in court for his troubles, charged with verbally abusing the morally ambiguous Mrs Brewster with obscene language. The situation was ideal material for shaping into a sensational journalistic narrative and the *Lincolnshire Chronicle* duly obliged, even including the deathbed terrors of the poor girl, who allegedly cried out somewhat melodramatically, 'Dying, dying, dying, I shall die, die, die.' The story contained additional interest in that the vermin poison had been purchased by Mildred Pepper from Battle's own shop on the High Street in Lincoln, accompanied by thirteen year old Lucy Hodson, who confirmed that her friend had purchased the product under the pretence of intending to keep it in a cupboard to kill mice.

Interestingly, but not surprisingly, the Lincoln surgeon, Dr Thomas Sympson, told the coroner's court that he had seen quite a few cases of death resulting from the consumption of *Battle's Vermin Killer* and was therefore able to confirm his verdict that Mildred Pepper had died from the ingestion of strychnine poison. The glib conclusion of the coroner, Mr Septimus Lowe, was that the young girl's mind had probably become unhinged after her father's remonstrations concerning her 'irregular habits', and feeling miserable, she had taken her own life. He directed the jury towards a verdict of temporary insanity, but not before making it clear that the packet of vermin killer found under Mildred Pepper's pillow had been clearly and responsibly labelled with the word 'Poison' – a fact which happily avoided any potential anxiety for John Richard Battle, alderman, former mayor of Lincoln and the joint owner of a thriving business in dangerous substances.

The jury followed the advice of the coroner.

The number of men buying *Battle's Vermin Killer* to end their troubles, compared to women, seems to have been comparatively low, although there may have been unrecorded cases at inquests where a specific vermin killer was either not named, not identified or could not be distinguished. The latter was evidently the case in Lincoln, on the 26th October, 1874, at the inquest into the death of Henry Harris, a merchant's clerk, where Dr George Lowe, the county analyst, admitted being unable to distinguish between *Butler's Vermin Killer* and *Battle's Vermin Killer*, as both used a similar blue colouring.

Unsuccessful suicide attempts, especially by obscure agricultural workers, tended to receive little notice in the popular press, beyond a brief paragraph which explained very little. Frederick Wilkinson, a labourer of Navenby appeared at the Kesteven Petty Sessions, in Lincoln, in March, 1881, for example, charged with attempted suicide after having purchased a packet of *Battle's Vermin Killer*. The short report in the *Lincolnshire Chronicle* suggested that Mr Wilkinson and his wife had been living on 'uncomfortable terms', whilst an earlier report on the case, published in the *Stamford Mercury,* provided a more scurrilous version of village gossip: Mrs Wilkinson had left her husband after a nasty altercation concerning the paternity of their son.

In court, Frederick Wilkinson expressed great contrition for his foolish act and was rewarded with a no-nonsense admonition from the Bench.

The suicide of George Richardson, a twenty-two year old baker of Market Rasen, in February, 1883, was reported more extensively by the newspapers: on the one hand, he had been successful in his shocking self-destruction, and on the other, there was a slightly scandalous backstory of romantic entanglement more usually associated with disreputable young women than respectable young men.

Mr Richardson was well known in the town and throughout the neighbourhood, and his death elicited great sympathy for his friends and family. The account of the unfortunate circumstances surrounding the tragedy, as reported in the *Lincolnshire Chronicle*, was a skilful compound of information, amateur psychology and melodrama.

George Richardson was allegedly 'very susceptible

to excitement' and his excitable character seemed to have been particularly tested when Miss Jane Shelton, a barmaid at the Gordon Arms on Queen Street, wrote him a letter wishing to end their relationship. Several letters and one unpleasant confrontation later, George Richardson bought a packet of *Battle's Vermin Killer* from Henry Payne, the nearby chemist, also on Queen Street, mixed it with water and drank it. He died in great agony at his home, but not before confiding to his sister, Mary Jane Richardson, 'it's that girl that's killed me.'

Predictably, the coroner's jury concluded that George Richardson had 'poisoned himself with strychnia whilst in a fit of temporary insanity'.

The passing comments of various Lincolnshire coroners and surgeons in the second half of the nineteenth century underline the continued alarming misuse of *Battle's Vermin Killer*, but the number of reported incidents between March 1870 and May 1871, mainly in the north of the county, was astonishing. It was a remarkable pattern which compelled Dr Sharpley, the coroner who had dealt with the cases, to comment upon it. His observation that there seemed to be a 'tendency' towards 'imitation in the means selected for committing suicide' was cautious and discreet, but there is a sense that he was avoiding having to voice the very worrying and sensational conclusion that there was an uncomfortable issue of emulation suicide in the area.

His concerns seemed justified.

On the 16th March, 1870, Mary Jane Robinson of Upton, a domestic servant in the employment of Thorpe Auctioneers, Gainsborough, killed herself with a sixpenny packet of *Battle's Vermin Killer*, seemingly after a quarrel with her young man, Enoch Brown. The inquest at the Ship Inn, recorded that she had written various letters, including one requesting that the photograph of Mr Brown should be placed in her coffin. Mr Brown, a man unencumbered by any inconvenient delicate feelings, did not emerge from the melancholy episode in a good light, testifying without any hint of regret that Mary Robinson had written him a letter the previous week which had contained the word 'poison' and that he had instantly burnt it. In addition, Charlotte Tyson, the cousin of Mary Robinson, gave evidence that Enoch Wood had left her and had 'behaved very badly'.

The declaration of Mary Jane Robinson in one of her final letters that 'I cannot bear the trouble any longer in this world' was an all too familiar echoing sound of despair.

Three weeks later, a similar bleak note was struck in Louth when Rebecca Hill, a widow and mother of three children, aged eight, eleven and thirteen, wrote in a suicide letter to her two friends, 'I seem quite beat out with everything I do', before swallowing

Battle's Vermin Killer. The narrative thread emerging from the inquest was a tangled one of a quite difficult woman, described as 'a dangerous person with her tongue', but at the end of her tether. Employed as a cleaner at Louth Town Hall, who occasionally took in sewing to supplement her £20 per annum income, Mrs Hill had found the sudden withdrawal of parish relief difficult. Her suicide, propelled by economic problems and a sense of grievance at perceived ill-treatment by her employers, seemed to have been carefully planned in that when she bought the vermin killer from the chemist shop of John Tatum Greenwood, located at 22 Market Place, Louth, and signed the *Poison Register* with a cross, having claimed to be illiterate.

John Greenwood was clear that Rebecca Hill had bought the vermin killer to kill mice; that the packet was properly labelled with the word 'Poison' and that he had responsibly entered the details of the transaction into his book.

The body of Rebecca Hill was discovered on a bed by her children, next to a table on which was found the tell-tale empty packet of *Battle's Vermin Killer*.

After a respite of only a few weeks, Dr Sharpley was once again required to preside over an inquest into the suicide of a young woman after swallowing *Battle's Vermin Killer*, this time at Sturton. Eliza Jane Graves, housekeeper to farmers George and Thomas

Scholey, had appeared to have been 'much depressed in spirits'. She had confessed to her employers to having consumed mice poison, before eventually dying in the early hours of the following morning. There was no mention of financial hardship or personal difficulties with a young man at the inquest, but the death of the young woman was no less shocking for having no clear motive to explain away such a desperate act of self-destruction.

In the terms of journalistic cliché, the appalling deaths of Mary Jane Robinson, Eliza Ann Graves and Rebecca Hill had caused 'great excitement". In the case of Sarah Ann Graves, a cook employed by Grimsby surgeon, George Holland JP, great excitement turned into a full scale riot in response to the unfolding horrors.

At the inquest into the suicide of the twenty-five year old in Louth, on the 9th May, 1871, it emerged that she had previously appeared in front of the magistrate several months earlier, accused of stealing meat from Samuel Topliss, a draper located on Mercer Row, Louth, who had employed her as a domestic servant. More recently, she had been accused by her employer, Dr George Holland, of stealing a postage stamp, for which she was found Guilty and sentenced to a day in prison, despite her protestations of innocence.

Worse still was to come for Sarah Ann Graves which probably contributed to her decision to seek solace in a packet of vermin killer.

In an attempt to find a new situation by using the Lincolnshire Registry Office of Mrs Matilda Brogden, located on Eastgate, in Louth, she discovered that she had been blacklisted on the advice of her former employer, Mrs Holland, who had recommended that Sarah Ann Graves be taken off the books. At the inquest, the plain-speaking Mrs Brogden testified that the deceased had asked her for a reference, but 'of course' she had declined. Further, she had spoken with her young man, who had read about the theft of the postage stamp in the newspapers, and had consequently decided that he was 'done with her': 'so have I', was Mrs Brogden's laconic, but empathetic reply to the morally upright young man. In a transparent piece of self-exoneration, the worthy lady assured the coroner's court that she had not noticed anything in particular about the reaction of Sarah Ann Graves when being refused a reference, and that even after she had reported the words of her young man to her, 'it did not seem to make any difference in her manner'.

Preferring a couple of hours of agony to a perceived lifetime of poverty and shame, Sarah Ann Graves bought a packet of *Battle's Vermin Killer* from the chemist shop of John Woodrow Dennis, on Eastgate, quite close to Mrs Brogden's office. Remarkably, Charles Richard Curry, the chemist's assistant, was as uncertain as to which young woman he had sold the poison, as Mrs Brogden was certain that she had followed the correct course of action in turning her away.

Dr Sharpley had no doubt as to the cause of death, but added that it was very probable that 'the news communicated to her by Mrs Brogden would drive her to despair': it was not clear whether he was referring to her being removed from the register or being rejected by her young man, or both. It may have been a coincidence, but the newspaper adverts for Mrs Brogden's Lincolnshire Registry Office ('The Oldest Established Registry Office in the Town and District') published after this date cautioned the reader that 'No servant with a known bad character will be registered'.

Summing up, Dr Sharpley lamented the fact that the sorry case of a young woman killing herself at a comparatively early age was the fifth he had dealt with over the last thirteen months.

With these sobering words and the interment of Sarah Ann Graves in Louth, the story of yet another distressed young woman destroying herself with *Battle's Vermin Killer* in North Lincolnshire seemed to have come to an end.

Unfortunately for Dr George Holland, it was not quite the case, as the outraged citizens of Grimsby, estimated to have been around ten thousand in number, but in reality probably far fewer than that, decided to share their understanding of the concept of fair play by taking to the streets in protest about what became known locally as 'The Postage Stamp Case'.

The demonstration took place between 8 o'clock on the evening of 19th May and around 1 o'clock the following morning, and was variously described as 'a procession', 'a disorderly proceeding' or 'a riot', depending upon which newspaper you read.

The conservative *Derbyshire Times and Chesterfield Herald* of 20th May, 1871 was surprisingly restrained, focusing upon factual details of the protest not reported in any Lincolnshire publications. Beyond the matter of fact observation that the huge crowd consisted mainly of fishermen and the working classes, there was little sense of any political analysis of a very volatile situation. Instead, it provided engaging descriptions of what was seen and heard on the streets, as the crowd moved inexorably towards the house of George Holland, clearly intent on mischief. The description in the newspaper created a sense of a holiday carnival occasionally on the edge of disorder, rather than a rampant mob storming through the streets of Grimsby.

The initial procession was accompanied by a band playing the *Dead March* from Handel's *Saul*, plus the popular song, *Poor Mary Ann*, as the crowd numbers gradually swelled along Cleethorpes Road. Numerous effigies accompanied the march, notably one covered with used postage stamps, mounted on a donkey and preceded by six tar barrels, which were later set alight on the common ground near Orwell Street 'amidst groans and execrations'. A wagon contained a tableau of young women symbolically guarding a young girl who represented Sarah Ann Graves; it also carried a large placard containing the words *Battle's Vermin Killer*, plus a satiric effigy labelled 'Dr Doodle'. The description was detailed, albeit a little muddled, in that the effigy covered in stamps was that of Dr Holland, which was eventually torched.

Almost inevitably, in view of the popular hostility and the lack of preparedness by the authorities, the house of Dr Holland on New Street was subjected to a violent attack in which over thirty plate-glass windows were smashed and the occupants intimidated with hoots and yells.

In the view of the reporter, the local authorities 'were quite powerless to prevent the noisy proceedings.'

The story of the 'Grimsby riot' was reported in London and various provincial newspapers, including the *Stamford Mercury* and the *Grantham Journal*, but mainly duplicated a widely circulated synoptic paragraph. The report in the ultra-Conservative *Lincolnshire Chronicle*, however, was much more extensive, offering its readers well over a thousand words of detailed background information, an account of the events which had taken place and a range of uncompromising opinions on those events.

From the outset, the main intention of the report was clear: it was an apoplectic declaration of outrage that a lawless attack on both person and property by a 'brutal rabble' should have taken place unchecked – specifically on such a worthy person of Mr George Holland, 'surgeon, magistrate, member of Grimsby Town Council and the Local Board of Health, and a gentlemen well-known in different parts of the county'.

On the one hand, the newspaper denigrated the protest as 'a foolish farce' and a mere 'puppet show', whilst on the other, it claimed that the streets of Grimsby had resembled the worst excesses of the Paris Commune: the mob violence and planned lawlessness were without doubt 'a collision of port and town'. The reporter was similarly unhelpful in his dark insinuations that the unrest had been deliberately orchestrated by conspirators who a few days earlier had distributed seditious prints intended to promulgate 'inflammatory, untruthful and sensational' material in order to arouse popular indignation against George Holland. The realities of what had led to the riot, 'where it was concocted, whence it came, or where, by an adjourned meeting, the organisation was completed', were well-known, the newspaper claimed, although without revealing to any puzzled reader what he or she was supposed to already know.

All he would say was that libel action and public prosecution would assuredly follow, in order to punish the guilty and to 'uncover what is hidden'; the *Stamford Mercury* was even more direct, declaring that the instigators of the outrage, who were apparently already known to the authorities, 'will be made to suffer for their folly'.

The stalwart defence of George Holland by the *Lincolnshire Chronicle* was further supported by a lame and partial recollection of his dealings with Sarah Ann Graves before her death.

The master had confronted his cook with the theft of a stamp and had been willing to let her go unpunished had she not had the temerity to deny the accusation and try to implicate other servants. 'No sensible man would expose himself to the possibility of being charged by a servant with having brought a false accusation against her', the report asserted, as a self-evident universal truth. She was therefore arrested and brought before the magistrates, and after an adjournment, was found guilty. Not only was impartial justice done, but also great indulgence had been shown towards the culprit by Dr Holland, who had only pressed for a formal conviction and one day in prison. Even more to the point, there was no prison in Grimsby, so the woman was never even detained and so had got off lightly.

The distressing death of Sarah Ann Graves was barely mentioned and when it was there was a sense of the reporter attempting to put some distance between the suicide and Dr and Mrs Holland. On leaving Grimsby for Louth on the day of her release, she was clearly not contemplating any act of self-destruction, as she had allegedly bought some new clothes from a draper's shop. The truth of the matter was that it was only after being told that she was being removed from the employment register and that her young man did not want anything more to do with her, that she came to a 'fatal resolution to destroy herself'. Significantly, no mention was made of a letter written by Mrs Holland to Mrs Brogden, which in effect removed any prospect of gaining useful employment in the area.

It was claimed that an alternative narrative of these events was being circulated in the area, which the reporter characterised as 'a gross misstatement of all the facts', promulgated by a 'busybody', and published in various editions of the mischievous print which had been doing the rounds in the town.

There seems little doubt that such a print did exist and was still circulating in the area for a short time afterwards.

Just two weeks after the disturbance, a curious

case of two 'tramping ballad singers' was reported in the *Lincolnshire Chronicle* who had crossed the borough boundary from Louth to Grimsby, and were apprehended by PC Clarke for hawking without permission. The two itinerant rascals had been caught going from door to door trying to sell copies of a song titled *Lines on the Lamentations of Sarah Graves*, no doubt offering added value to any purchase with an engaging rendition.

Appearing before a Grimsby magistrate, the unnamed pair of likely lads claimed that they had been given two hundred copies of the printed verses by a mysterious 'tall gentleman', near the railway bridge, and that they had sold over half of them. In their defence, but somewhat disingenuously, they 'understood the verses had a local significance, but thought they could hawk them as they pleased'.

The magistrate strongly disagreed and discharged the pair on payment of six shillings and sixpence each in order to cover the expenses of the court, which probably wiped out their pre-arrest profits.

The media coverage of the suicide of Sarah Ann Graves and its surrounding circumstances seemed to fizzle out with the *Lincolnshire Chronicle* report of the attack on the house of George Holland. In general, the newspapers had dutifully expressed dismay at the death of the young woman, but were uncritical of the conduct of her employers and their associates. The most sympathetic report on the case was probably that found in *Reynold's Newspaper*, published on 21st May, which described the story of Sarah Ann Graves as 'a truly melancholic one' and highlighted the strong condemnation of Mrs Brogden by Dr Sharpley 'for telling the poor woman that her young man had given her up'.

After reading the account of the Grimsby riot in the *Lincolnshire Chronicle*, George Holland may well have sat back and breathed a sigh of relief that the influential county newspaper had rallied round and exonerated him from any wrongdoing.

If he had read the substantial feature article published in the *Illustrated Police News*, on the 27th May, however, any such complacency would have very quickly evaporated. The London newspaper with a reputation for sensationalist reporting and an undisguised populist agenda reported on the demonstration in Grimsby in support of Sarah Ann Graves: it was a complete contrast with that published in the *Lincolnshire Chronicle* and was clearly intent on publicly exposing those whom it thought responsible for her suicide.

Having a copy of the newspaper to hand, he would also have been aghast to discover that he was front page news, alongside the appalling murder of seventeen-year old Jane Clouson, who had been bludgeoned to death with a hammer in Eltham. Even worse, there was a graphic illustration of Dr Holland's house under attack, and below it a second image, depicting a grotesque comic effigy of him, mounted on a cart and holding a large sheet of postage stamps stuck on a stick.

Whilst a degree of scepticism should be applied to the absolute truthfulness of the account, it is a useful counterbalance to that published in the *Lincolnshire Chronicle*.

The newspaper began its disapproval by noting that at the trial of Sarah Ann Graves, brought before the magistrates on a 'frivolous charge' of stealing a postage stamp, Dr Holland had taken up his position on the Bench and, at the same time, had given evidence against her, much to the consternation of some of the public who were observing the court proceedings.

Whilst making it clear that the newspaper 'strongly condemned the manner in which the Grimsby friends and sympathisers of the unfortunate girl have displayed their feelings against Mr Holland', it also insisted that 'he can scarcely be deemed blameless for the somewhat unseemly position he occupied'.

After reminding its readers of the progress of universal literacy, the introduction of 'cheap and well-regulated newspapers' and the growing importance of the vox populi, the article maintained that the procession at Grimsby was not 'a reckless mob of roughs': on the contrary, it consisted of many law-abiding and respectable citizens. It was an easy claim to make, but the precision of the references to the local area in its tracking of the progress of the march towards the house of Dr Holland suggested that the report was making use of reliable local sources on the ground.

Similarly, the understated information, not included in any other newspaper report, that Dr Holland had 'kept watch and ward' outside his house until forced to retreat from the missiles which were being thrown at the windows, suggested an authenticity beyond dramatic invention. The additional information that Mrs Holland, an invalid, was removed for her own safety from the premises to the residence of Edward Bannister, the former mayor, seemed also to confirm the use of well-informed eye-witnesses. In a spirit of journalistic gallantry, the reporter rejoiced that Mrs Holland, a woman of exemplary life, had been protected from insult and injury. The characterisation of Mrs Holland as having led a totally blameless life, of course, chose to ignore the impact on Sarah Ann Graves of having been blacklisted by Mrs Brogden in her obsequious acceptance of the letter advising her removal from the employment register.

The report concluded on a sympathetic note concerning the lack of effective policing. The constabulary had been powerless to prevent the destruction of property, it was true, but had been completely outnumbered. 'What could they do against a mass of 7,000 or 8,000 people in possession of every thoroughfare around the residence?', the reporter asked rhetorically: it seemed a fair point.

In order to either support its account of the incident, or to create the illusion of impartiality, the *Illustrated Police News* appended a version of the story taken from an unnamed local newspaper. Essentially, it provided more precise location details of the progress of the march from near the Ebenezer Chapel in New Clee to the house of George Holland, and further modified the claim in the *Lincolnshire Chronicle* of extensive violent disorder on the streets of Grimsby. On the contrary, the procession 'passed off most orderly', at least until it reached the home of Dr Holland, who was standing outside his door, intending to 'brave the matter out'. At this point, the demonstrators became an 'enraged mob', and proceeded to 'manifest their displeasure at his conduct', by throwing stones and smashing thirty windows. There would have been worse, the newspaper thought, had the angry crowd not been restrained by the knowledge that Mrs Holland was in the house 'suffering from a disease which has recently been so fatal in the town'. The infectious disease in question was almost certainly the outbreak of smallpox, which had been reported in early April, and had lately impacted on the new part of the town where Dr and Mrs Holland lived.

The newspaper, in the final analysis, expressed its wish to be impartial, leaving the public 'to judge for themselves on the merits and demerits of the case'. However, there was a clear sense where its sympathies lay when it highlighted the 'thoroughly English' feelings which had prompted the leaders of the demonstration to give expression to popular opinion.

In a final contrast to the threat and bluster of the *Lincolnshire Chronicle* and the *Stamford Mercury*, the article concluded that 'nothing further will arise out of the affair', now that public feeling against 'the principal character in the drama' had been vented.

The account, vaguely described as 'a supplement to one of the local newspapers' by the *Illustrated Police News,* is curious in that it makes no mention of the part played by Matilda Brogden in the unfolding story. Even more curious, perhaps, is that Frederic William Brogden, her husband, was involved in the world of local journalism by way of being an agent for the *Lincoln Gazette* and also being the publisher, every Tuesday, of the *Lincolnshire Halfpenny Echo*, from his residence on Eastgate, a few years later.

It was a melancholy and remarkable postscript to the suicide of Sarah Ann Graves, two months later, when Dr Sharpley conducted an inquest into the death of Frederick William Brogden at Louth, aged sixteen, suspected of drowning himself in the canal. The newspaper reports of the time recorded strenuous efforts by his father, Frederick Brogden, to establish a sense of domestic harmony and the boy having no reason to take his own life. In the end, the verdict was an uncontentious one of Death by Drowning, despite pieces of unresolved circumstantial evidence, which included a scribbled note begging forgiveness from his mother and father; in addition, some of the jury had heard of domestic difficulties at the time – something 'distinctly denied' by the dead boy's father.

Not unlike the case of Sarah Ann Graves, it was a reconstructed narrative of the heart-breaking suicide of a young person, fraught with ambiguity and uneasiness, but apparently resolved into a convenient certainty.

The astonishing unintended social consequences resulting from the suicide of a desperate young woman from Alvingham, using *Battle's Vermin Killer* to end her troubles, like the concerned words of Professor Swaine Taylor, seemed to have little significant impact in terms of addressing uncomfortable questions, halting the horror or facing up to responsibilities.

Despite the number of insistent alerts from juries to presiding judges and coroners concerning the continued irresponsibility or carelessness of chemists as a significant factor in poisoning cases, and the annus horribilis of March, 1870 to May, 1871 having been flagged up by Dr Sharpley, little seemed to change in terms of the reckless selling and misuse of vermin killer in the county.

In March, 1879, Crowle chemist John Sharpe, was fined ten shillings plus costs, for selling *Battle's Vermin Killer* without making an entry in his book and for failing to ask the name of purchaser, who unfortunately for Mr Sharpe, happened to be a policeman. In January, 1881, Nathaniel Boon, a chemist in Ashby, was also heavily fined, for having sold *Battle's Vermin Killer* without having written his name and address on the packet. A year later, in May, 1882, Mr Utterby Boles, an agricultural labourer from Algarkirk, was summoned to appear at the Boston Sessions House for his freelance selling of vermin killer. The entrepreneurial Mr Boles had purchased what was probably *Battle's Vermin Killer* from a local chemist, completely removed the wrapper and re-sold it. In his defence, the unofficial dealer in dangerous substances, claimed that he did not make any profit nor meant to do any harm. Probably more out of pity at his incompetence as a petty criminal than as an act of judicial retribution, the charge against the redoubtable Mr Boles was withdrawn on payment of court costs.

Whilst the unlawful activities of Utterby Boles

did not seem to have had any serious consequences, such an ingrained cavalier attitude to the handling of vermin killer was still producing fatal consequences in small rural communities.

The practice of coating pieces of bread with vermin killer, for example, seemed to have continued as a commonplace of pest control, based upon traditional domestic practices. Unfortunately, it was also potentially a commonplace of accidental poisoning. In January, 1883, the *Grantham Journal* reported the death of two young children in Dairycoates, near Hull, after playing out with their friends. The verdict of the inquest was that they had been poisoned by eating either poisonous herbs or more probably, bread and butter coated with *Battle's Vermin Killer*.

In 1889, Sheffield-based Dr Alfred Allen presented a paper at the British Pharmaceutical Conference in Newcastle, which strongly suggested that the anxieties of Professor Swaine Taylor concerning the easy and slip-shod availability of strychnine-based vermin killer, were still depressingly relevant over thirty years later.

An interest in the subject had grown out of his involvement as an expert medical witness in the case of eight-year old Kate Horton, from the village of Swanwick in Derbyshire, who had died in suspicious circumstances. The life of the young girl had been insured by her father and after conviction he had confessed to having emptied vermin killer into a bottle and given it to his daughter to drink.

Allen had examined the viscera of Kate Horton, identified the presence of strychnine and made a telling contribution to uncovering the horrific crime. However, his interest went beyond the medical formalities of an inquest, in that he became aware of the significant part played by local pharmacists in the accidental and intentional misuse of vermin killer. His research suggested that whilst pharmacists sold a wide range of commercial vermin killers, the majority preferred to make up their own powder. His analysis of a number of these powders showed that the colouring in them, on the whole, was ultramarine, which in his opinion was inadequate in terms of ensuring visibility and attracting the attention of the taker.

His recommendation was that a more effective pigment would be chrome green, which had the added advantage of not being destroyed by cremating the body.

In words reminiscent of those used by Swaine Taylor in 1864, Alfred Allen also insisted that shops selling strychnine-based products should 'take more care to record sales of vermin killer in the poison book than was at present the practice in some districts'.

A report on Allen's paper was published in the *Sheffield Daily Telegraph*, 30th July, 1889, but only provided a brief synopsis of its content. What it did not show was important data related to various commercial vermin killers, as well as a useful list of their names. The tabular information published in the *Pharmaceutical Journal*, 12th October, 1889, was helpful in terms of a comparative study of the contents of commercial and local preparations.

It was also interesting in its analysis of *Battle's Vermin Killer* in that it observed that the Lincoln product was 'probably the best known and most extensively used', but over time its composition had changed and that it had 'varied in other periods' – an observation which may have had retrospective implications for some inquest judgements.

Despite accidents waiting to happen, or actually happening, casual malpractice continued towards the end of the century in the use of vermin killers. The directions for the use of *Carlton's Vermin Killer*, a short lived product sold in Horncastle and Woodhall Spa, which were regularly published in the *Horncastle News and South Lindsey Advertiser* in the first half of 1897, for example, seemed oblivious to the dangers of its instructions. The recommended way to kill mice might have been found in any eighteenth century book on vermin destruction: 'Sprinkle a small quantity of the killer on thin pieces of bread and butter, or bread covered with bacon grease, cut into pieces about an inch square, and lay in the most frequented places'.

The directions did not mention any potential hazards to small hungry children, but thoughtfully insisted that cats and dogs should be kept well away from it.

Whilst some small shops continued to flout the strict rules relating to the sale of vermin killer, perhaps under the perceived cover of rural obscurity, the most prominent commercial enterprise in Lincolnshire found itself in serious hot water in 1896: Battle, Son & Maltby, inventors and purveyors of *Battle's Vermin Killer*, were summoned by the Lincoln City Police to explain certain irregular commercial transactions.

It wasn't the first embarrassing mishap which had befallen the Lincoln shop. In 1852, Mrs Hill, the lady mayoress, thought that she had been sold Rochelle Salts, a mild aperient, but instead she had been given the rather more aggressive Tartar Emetic, resulting in her vomiting and being seized with violent pains. Described by the *Lincolnshire Chronicle* as 'a lamentable error' and 'an unfortunate affair', which had apparently also given Mr Battle 'great pain', the apprentice who had served Mrs Hill, was dismissed on the spot.

The latest unfortunate mistake was rather more high profile than the severe discomfort of the lady mayoress of Lincoln, as it involved the Pharmaceutical Society of Great Britain accusing the Lincoln company of two separate, but related offences. Contrary to the 1868 *Pharmaceutical Act*, a product containing strychnine had been sold to a person who was not known to the shop, and in addition, the packet was in several respects inadequately labelled.

In court, the Society was represented by Mr R E Vaughan-Williams of London, and Battle, Son & Maltby by Mr J G Williams of Lincoln.

The first charge related to a Mr Moon of Brocklesby who had written to the shop for a packet of *Battle's Vermin Killer*, which had been posted out to him the following day. The second sale was rather more damning in that Mr Foulds of Manchester, employed by the Pharmaceutical Society of Great Britain as an enquiry agent, had managed to buy the vermin killer over the counter: he had been asked to sign his name against the sale, but was not previously known as a customer.

The arguments presented in court, as reported by the *Stamford Mercury,* were low key. On the first charge, the Prosecution witnesses, Mr Foulds and Mr Moon, confirmed that they had been sold the vermin killer without being known to the shop. On the second charge, the Prosecution acknowledged that the vermin killer was contained in three wrappers within a sealed envelope with 'Battle's Vermin Killer' on the front and the word 'Poison' on the reverse. However, Mr Vaughan-Williams contended that the packet of poison did not have sufficient wording to show 'who was the actual seller and what was his proper address'. On both counts, he suggested, there had been a serious infringement of the regulations.

For the Defence, Mr Williams, agreed with the description of the wording on the sealed envelope, but also pointed out that the words 'Battle, Lincoln' were printed on the inside wrapper. The charge of selling strychnine to an unknown party was more difficult to dispute and the Defence fell back on the feeble argument that this constituted only 'the slightest technical offence'. That such technical offences sometimes led to tragedy, as in the case of sixteen year-old Mildred Pepper when she was sold *Battle's Vermin Killer* at the shop, in 1883, was not mentioned.

In a spirit of compromise, it seems, the Bench dismissed the charge of inadequate labelling, but upheld that of selling to unknown persons. The law was partially vindicated and the commercial reputation of Battle, Sons & Maltby was partially rescued.

The extent to which *Battle's Vermin Killer* had become embedded in the popular nineteenth century consciousness as a dispenser of death and destruction is evident from specific references to it in contexts other than suicide, murder and commercial enterprise. In the middle of a libel trial, contested between Messrs Hole and Co, brewers of Newark, and Mr John Richardson, JP, of Lincoln, in March

1892, Justice Sir John Lawrance, prompted by the mere mention of the word 'vermin' by the Learned Counsel, dryly observed that '*Battle's Vermin Killer* is well-known all over Lincolnshire': a comment which prompted some knowing, but possible uneasy laughter in the courtroom. Five years later, in a letter to the editor of the *Lincolnshire Echo*, an irate rate payer, clearly lacking good will to all men, proposed that the 'can work, but won't work brigade', currently resident in the Union Workhouse, should not be served with a Christmas dinner, but rather less charitably, with 'a good dose of *Battle's Vermin Killer*'.

The product was still being advertised and sold by chemists well into the first half of the twentieth-century, but had its fleeting apotheosis in the speculative suggestion that Glydmr Michael, a tramp whose dead body was used in a deception operation by British Intelligence in 1943, codenamed *Mincemeat*, had committed suicide using *Battle's Vermin Killer*, before being quietly recruited as part of the war effort in mainland Europe.

DISPENSING DEATH AND DESTRUCTION FOR ONLY A FEW PENCE

Particulars of the sales of all substances included in the FIRST SCHEDULE to the RULES required to be

Date of sale	Name and quantity of poison supplied	Purchaser's Name	Purchaser's Address	Business, trade or occupation
21.10.40	1 Beaker, 1 Zinc Balls, 1 B.Q.	C.S. Chown	5 Stephenson's Road	[illegible]
5.11.40	1×5" Bottle Vermin Killer	Mr. T. Hinton	8 Oath Road	Shopkeeper
5.11.40	1×1ℓ Auto Fluids	G. Liddall	54 Manor Rd, Barnstaple	[illegible]
6.11.40	6. Engel Expander gas	Three Seniors	2 Albernus Road	[illegible]
26.11.40	3oz Inst. Essence Opio...	Mr. Prior	56 Invin St.	[illegible]
25.11.40	[illegible]	Mrs. [illegible]	137 Water Rd.	Mrs.
6.12.40	4 ozs Emerald Green	W. H. Lyell	18 Woolsworth St	[illegible]
9.12.40.	10ℓ Auto Sprinkle	T. Johnson	29 Greenfield Avenue	[illegible]
3.1.41	[illegible] Vermin [illegible]	Mr. Nuttall	19 The Rd	[illegible]
28.1.41.	2gℓ In. A.B.C.	Mrs. Conhight	23 Clement Kings Bottom	[illegible]
18.2.41	1q Ung Gallow i Opio	Mr. J. Evans	84 Queen St.	Retired
24.2.41	2oz Ung Gallae i Opio	Mr. Burke	36 Queen St.	[illegible]

APPENDIX

List of 19th Century Vermin Killers

The list below records the name of the main commercial vermin killers available in nineteenth century England, along with information relating to their sale and distribution. The short extracts from newspaper accounts of inquests and trials focus upon some of the issues relating to the misuse and maladministration of vermin killers, which were mentioned by Alfred Swaine Taylor, in 1864, and were still being highlighted a quarter of a century later by Alfred Allen.

Any reference to an advert for a particular vermin killer is the earliest which I have been able to find and is included as an estimated date for the product's initial availability on the market.

Those products annotated with the name of Alfred Allen refer to vermin killers listed by him in the paper delivered at the British Pharmaceutical Conference, at Newcastle, in 1889.

PRODUCT
Adshead's Infallible Vermin and Insect Killer

ORIGIN OF PRODUCT
William Peter Adshead, chemist, Belper, Derbyshire.

NOTES
Advert: *Bury Free Press*, 18th December, 1869. p.8.

Adshead's Rat Poison.

ONE SMALL POT has been known to KILL 20 STRONG RATS in a single night. It is easy to use, and not so dangerous as other preparations.

Misuse
Trial of Martha Calladine of Heanor, accused of poisoning her husband, held at the Derbyshire Assizes, 3rd March, 1870. Prisoner found Guilty and sentenced to fourteen years penal servitude.

'Mr. William Adshead, manufacturing chemist, Belper, said the poison in the packets contained strychnine. Mr. Frederick Chapman, druggist, Heanor, said that he had sold the prisoner a twopenny packet of vermin killer on the 22nd October, supplied to him by Mr. Greaves, of Chesterfield. She stated that she had many mice in her house'.

Source: *Sheffield Daily Telegraph*, 5th March, 1870, p.3.

PRODUCT
Barber's Magic Vermin Killer

ORIGIN OF PRODUCT
Barber's Poisoned Wheat Works, Butter Market, Ipswich.

NOTES
Listed by Alfred Allen.

Advert: *Suffolk Chronicle*, 29th August, 1863, p.2.

Kills Rats and Mice. Mice tumble over, and die on the spot by hundreds. In Packets 2d, 3d, 6d and 1s.

Misuse
Trial at Norwich of Henry Grimstone, fifty-two, itinerant fiddler, charged with attempting to inflict grievous bodily harm on Ann Grimstone, his wife, with *Barber's Magic Vermin Killer*. Acquitted.

Source: *Norwich Mercury*, 23rd June, 1869, p.3.

The Dudley Poisoning Case. Trial of Fanny Oliver, milliner, twenty-eight, of Dudley, accused of poisoning her husband, Joseph Oliver, held at Worcester County and City Assizes, 21st July, 1869. Prisoner found Guilty, but with a recommendation for mercy. Reprieved from death sentence, 2nd August, 1869, commuted to penal servitude for life.

William George Vose deposed: 'I am a chemist and a druggist, in Dudley Street, Brierley Hill, close to Dudley....I sell some powder for killing mice. It is called *Barber's vermin destroyer*, or *vermin killer*. I didn't remember selling any of it to Annie Archer until the prisoner was taken. She came with a police officer. I don't remember selling her any before that'.

Source: Supplement to *Worcester Chronicle*, 21st July, 1869, pp.5-6.

Dr Alfred Hill, Professor of Chemistry and Toxicology at Queen's College, Birmingham: 'Believed deceased had taken sufficient arsenic to cause death. When before the magistrates would not swear that the deceased died from arsenic poisoning. Witness would now swear to his positive conviction that deceased died from poisoning by arsenic. Considered that strychnine was not the cause of death, from the absence of tetanic convulsions and from the inflammation. The essential ingredient of Barber's vermin killer was strychnine. Did not test it for arsenic'.

Source: *Worcester Chronicle*, 24th July, 1869, p.7.

Inquest into the suicide of Emma Ordidge of Wednesbury, 8th November, 1869, twenty-three, married, three months pregnant, at the Talbot Inn, Wednesbury. Verdict: Temporary Insanity.

'The druggist stated that the deceased had been a customer of his for three years previous to purchasing the vermin killer on Friday. The sale on that day was registered, and deceased put her cross to his book. He noticed nothing unusual in her manner; but he always observed that she had a peculiar look in her eyes, and a wild look, though she always conversed rationally'.

Source: *Birmingham Daily Gazette*, 11th November, 1869, p.5.

PRODUCT
Bartlett's Magic Vermin Killer

ORIGIN OF PRODUCT
H Bartlett, Chemist and Dental Surgeon, 12 Market Place, Banbury.

NOTES
Advert: *Banbury Guardian*, 20th September, 1888, p.2.

MICE, RATS, MICE.
Houses, stacks, farm buildings, warehouses et cetera, are speedily cleared of Rats, Mice, Beetles, and other vermin, by *Bartlett's Magic Vermin Killer*, in Packets 3d, 6d and 1s.

PRODUCT
Battle's Vermin Killer

ORIGIN OF PRODUCT
J R Battle, Chemist, 294 High Street, Lincoln.

NOTES
Listed by Alfred Allen.

Advert: *Stamford Mercury*, 1st February, 1850, p.3

Houses, Stacks, Farm Buildings, Warehouses, Mills, et cetera, speedily cleared of Rats and Mice, by Battle's Vermin Killer. Mice eat it readily, and die on the spot.

Prepared only, and sold in Packets at 3d, 6d and 1s, by J R Battle, Chemist, Lincoln.

See text above *passim*.

PRODUCT
Board's Vermin Killer

ORIGIN OF PRODUCT
Thomas Board, Chemist, 317 High Street, Cheltenham.

NOTES
Advert: *Cheltenham Examiner*, 17th March, 1858, p.1.

Important to Farmers, Millowners, Shipmasters, Innkeepers and Housekeepers of all ranks, for the speedy destruction of RATS, MICE, BEETLES, BUGS, CRICKETS, and all other kind of vermin. Sold in packets 3d, 6d and 1s each, by the Proprietor, 317 High Street, opposite the old hospital.

PRODUCT
Brett's Vermin Killer

ORIGIN OF PRODUCT
Samuel Fisher Brett, Chemist, Queen Street, Market Rasen.

NOTES
Advert: *Nottingham Guardian*, 27th July, 1854, p.2.

An effectual and sure article for the destruction of Rats and Mice, in Houses, Warehouses, Corn Ricks, Farm Buildings et cetera.

Directions: In houses et cetera, a little of the powder to be sprinkled on thin bits of bread, or bread and butter, put them at night in the place most frequented by the vermin, and in the morning the mice will be found dead lying near the poison. Rats will generally die in their holes; great care should be taken so that nothing else can get to the poison.

PRODUCT
Brown's Vermin Killer

ORIGIN OF PRODUCT
John Brown, chemist, Market Square, Hanley.

NOTES
Misuse

Mary Ann Johnson, domestic servant, charged at Hanley Borough Magistrate's Court, 4th February, 1869, with attempting to commit suicide using *Brown's Vermin Killer*. Conditionally released on guarantee of her finding sureties for her good behaviour.

'Mr. Brown, chemist. Market-square, said that the prisoner called at his shop on the day in question, and asked for some rat poison for Mrs. Peake, of Shelton; and after questioning her, he supplied her with a packet of Vermin Killer, and registered it in his book. He said he had been informed by the Pharmaceutical Society that it was not necessary to restrict the sale of Vermin Killer. Mr. Baker called the attention of the Bench to the clause of the Act of Parliament which imposed the restriction, which certainly differed very materially from Mr. Brown's information'.

Source: The *Staffordshire Sentinel*, 6th February, 1869, p.6.

PRODUCT
Butler's Vermin Killer/ Butler's Vermin and Insect Killer/Butler's Gloucestershire Vermin and Insect Killer

ORIGIN OF PRODUCT
Wooton under Edge, Gloucestershire.

NOTES
Listed by Alfred Allen.

Advert: *Bristol Mercury*, 30th August, 1845, p.4.

LOSS AND DAMAGE PREVENTED – TO CAPTAINS & OWNERS OF VESSELS, FARMERS et cetera, et cetera.

The following striking testimonials of the success of *BUTLER'S GLOUCESTERSHIRE VERMIN AND INSECT KILLER*, in destroying rats and mice, renders interested praise needless.

The "Killer" is put up in packets, with full directions, at 3d, 6d and 1s each.

See text above *passim*.

PRODUCT
Carlton's Vermin Killer

ORIGIN OF PRODUCT
William Paston Carlton, Chemist and Druggist, High Street , Horncastle; later, Chemist and Photographer.

NOTES
Advert: *Horncastle News and South Lindsey Advertiser*, 9th January, 1897, p.4.

Granaries, Farm Buildings, Stacks, Warehouse, et cetera, et cetera, speedily cleared of mice and rats by *Carlton's Vermin Killer*.

They eat it readily and die on the spot.

Directions for use: 'Fish will be found almost the best bait, upon which the Killer may be sprinkled, and well pricked in with a fork. It is best to give the rats a treat of fish for a night or two before laying the Killer'.

PRODUCT
Casterton's Vermin Killer

ORIGIN OF PRODUCT
John Casterton, Queen Street, Market Rasen.

NOTES
Advert: *Market Rasen Weekly Mail*, 22nd March, 1862, p.1.

Casterton's Vermin Killer. Warranted to Kill. In packets at 3d and 6d.

PRODUCT
Clift's Magic Vermin Killer

NOTES
Listed by Alfred Allen.

Misuse
Attempted suicide at Woolwich by William Cook, solicitor's clerk, and a young man 'of dissipated appearance'. Swallowed a quantity of *Clift's Magic Vermin Killer* in a glass of beer, after resigning his position, deserting his wife and child and selling all his furniture.

Source: *The Kentish Independent*, 25th September, 1869. p.4.

'A druggist has been find half-a-crown, and costs at Bishop's Castle for selling a packet of *Clift's Magic Vermin Killer*, the same not being labelled with the name and address of the seller, with the word "Poison", and its description thereon'.

Source: *The Oswestry Chronicle and Montgomeryshire Mercury*, 26th January, 1870, p.7.

Suicide at Landport, Hampshire, of Sarah Jane Saunders, a married woman, who had been under of police supervision. Her daughter came home and found her ill. She asked if she had taken anything, but her mother denied it. On the discovery of an empty packet of *Clift's Magic Vermin Killer,* she admitted having swallowed the contents.

Source: *Hampshire Telegraph*, 26th January, 1876, p.2.

PRODUCT
Cowan's Magic Vermin Destroyer

ORIGIN OF PRODUCT
S A Cowan, London.

NOTES
Advert: *The Watford Observer*, 28th January, 1865, p.1.

The Great Discovery of the Age.

S A Cowan's Magic Vermin Destroyer.
This celebrated preparation is certain death to Black Beetles, Cockroaches, Crickets, Rats, and Mice. Thousands may be destroyed in one night without any danger to household Pets. In consequence of the immense demand, Agents have been appointed in every town in the United Kingdom.

PRODUCT
Cowin and Brahams' Magic Vermin Destroyer

NOTES
Advert: *The Rugby Advertiser*, 15th March, 1862, p.8.

This infallible Preparation is certain death to Rats,

Mice, Black Beetles, Cockroaches et cetera. Vermin eat it greedily and hundreds may be cleared in one night without danger to domestic animals.

PRODUCT
Craven's Vermin Killer

NOTES
Listed by Alfred Allen.

PRODUCT
Emery's Magic Beetle Poison

ORIGIN OF PRODUCT
C. Emery & Co , 35 Foley Place, London.

NOTES
Advert: *Bicester Advertiser*, 21st January, 1860, p.1.

Black Beetles, Cockroaches and Mice.

CERTAIN ANNIHILATION TO THESE DOMESTIC PESTS by using *EMERY'S BEETLE POISON*, well known as an effectual exterminator of these unwelcome intruders; possessing at the same time the inestimable property of freedom from danger to human life, and to cats and dogs.

PRODUCT
Fabin's Vermin Killer

ORIGIN OF PRODUCT
33 Carley Street, Lincoln's Inn, London.

NOTES
Advert: *The Bucks Herald*, 13th December, 1862, p.1.

Vermin! Vermin!!

Rats, mice, beetles, and cockroaches.

Over a million of either destroyed in forty-eight hours, by an outlay of 2d. Fabin's remedy is the only safe, but simple and never-failing one, recipe sent for twelve stamps and directed envelope. Address, Mr. Fabin, 33, Carley-street, Lincoln's Inn, London.

P.S.—One trial will prove the fact.

PRODUCT
Faulkner's Magic Vermin Powder

ORIGIN OF PRODUCT
R Faulkner, 12 Market Place, Banbury.

NOTES
Advert: *Banbury Guardian*, 1st January, 1880, p.4.

MICE, RATS, MICE

Houses, Stacks, Farm Buildings, Warehouses et cetera, are speedily cleared of Rats, Mice, Beetles and other Vermin by *Faulkner's Magic Vermin Killer*.

Sold in Packets of 3d, 6d and 1s.

PRODUCT
Fletcher's Infallible Vermin Killer

ORIGIN OF PRODUCT
The Office, 21 Basinghall Street, Leeds.

NOTES
Advert: *Leeds Times*, 2nd September, 1854, p.1.

FLETCHER'S INFALLIBLE VERMIN KILLER is the only certain means of destroying vermin. Its efficacy has been acknowledged by thousands of householders, both in town and country.

PRODUCT
Floyd's Vermin Killer

NOTES
Listed by Alfred Allen.

PRODUCT
Fowler's Vermin Killer

ORIGIN OF PRODUCT
William R Fowler, Pharmaceutical Chemist, 7 Market Place, Boston.

NOTES
Advert: *Boston Guardian*, 16th April, 1881, p.6.

A tempting killer of mice and rats, never failing to have the desired results. Price 3d, 6d and 1/-.

Misuse
Suicide: shoemaker, Isaac Jackson, resident at 8, Cheapside, Boston. 'Deceased, who was thirty six years of age, went to Mr Fowler's chemist's shop, in the Market Place, and purchased some vermin killer, which he swallowed'.

Source: *Lincolnshire Chronicle*, 30th January, 1883, p.3.

PRODUCT
Gibson's Vermin Killer

ORIGIN OF PRODUCT
Henry Atkin Gibson, Chemist, Market Place, Spalding; later, 18 Bridge Street.

NOTES
Listed by Alfred Allen.

Misuse
Accidental poisoning of child at Stalybridge. 'Elizabeth Ann Worthington, aged one year and eleven months…was accidentally poisoned by having a dose of *Gibson's vermin killer* administered to it. The child was teething, and on Monday morning, a woman who was nursing it gave the infant, with the consent of the mother, a dose of what was thought to be teething powder. Immediately on taking it the child was seized with convulsions, and died in a few minutes, and it was then discovered that they had administered powder for killing vermin. The package was properly labelled, but the woman could not read'.

Source: *Grantham Journal*, 30th July, 1870, p.7.

Attempted suicide. Sarah Peach, seventeen, domestic servant of Mr Palmer at the Lincoln Arms, Bridge Street, Spalding. 'It appears that on the morning in question, the girl went to the shop of Mr Asling, chemist, and asked for two ounces of laudanum, alleging that she required it for her face, which was swollen at the time. She was refused the quantity for which she asked, but was supplied with half an ounce of the poison. She then proceeded to Mr Gibson's, and bought a threepenny packet of *Gibson's Vermin Killer,* intimating that Mrs Palmer, her mistress, required it to kill mice with. She then returned to the Lincoln Arms, and at 12 o'clock took the laudanum. This not proving effectual, at 1 o'clock, she mixed up the vermin killer in a cup and swallowed it'.

Source: *Lincolnshire Free Press*, 15th March, 1881, p.3.

PRODUCT
Green's Infallible Vermin Killer/Green's Magic Vermin Killer

ORIGIN OF PRODUCT
John Green, High Street, Christchurch, near Bournemouth

NOTES
Advert: *The Christchurch Times*, 19th May 1877, p.4.

Green's Infallible Vermin Killer, for the DESTRUCTION of RATS and MICE, Speedily clears Houses, Warehouses, Farm Buildings, Stacks, Granaries etc, of the above Vermin, at the most trifling cost.

Misuse
Inquest on Albert Hammerton, Quartermaster-Sergeant, at the Town Hall, Christchurch. 'John Godwin Protheroe, chemist's assistant at Mr Green's, proved that he bought a threepenny packet of *Green's Vermin Killer* on the 7th April, and produced the book which he signed. He said it was for killing mice in the stores...Mr John Green deposed that the active principle in the vermin killer sold at his store is strychnine, of which there are two grains in a threepenny packet'.

Source: *Hampshire Independent*, 16th June, 1877, p.7.

PRODUCT
Greer's Anti-Vermin Preparations

ORIGIN OF PRODUCT
Robert Greer, 49 Brownlow Hill, Liverpool.

NOTES
Advert: *Liverpool Mercury and Lancashire, Cheshire General Advertiser*, 15th August, 1856, p.1.

An anti-vermin office is now established at 49 Brownlow Hill, conducted under the direction of Mr ROBERT GREER, one of the Liverpool Inspectors of Nuisances, for the sanitary object of furnishing the public with his newly discovered Chemical and Patented Materials, together with every requisite information, for the immediate and permanent EXTINCTION of all kinds of HOUSE and Land INSECTS and VERMIN.

PRODUCT
Griffith's Magic Vermin Killer

ORIGIN OF PRODUCT
G Griffith, Dispensing Chemist, High Street, Weston-super-Mare.

NOTES
Advert: *Weston-super-Mare Gazette and General Advertiser*, 13th December, 1862, p.7.

CERTAIN POISON FOR RATS!
(Woodcut of rat on pantry shelf, next to a block of cheese)

MAGIC VERMIN KILLER
This Preparation is confidently recommended as the best ever offered to the Public for the destruction of RATS and MICE. Mice are particularly attracted to it as if charmed, and die on the spot.

PRODUCT
Haines's Vermin Killer

ORIGIN OF PRODUCT
J Haines, Chemist, Market Place, Bromsgrove.

NOTES
Advert: *Bromsgrove and Droitwich Messenger*, 22nd March, 1862, p.1.

Vermin Killer for Destroying MICE and RATS.

PRODUCT
Hartley's Lancashire Vermin Killer

NOTES
Advert: *St Noet's Chronicle and Huntingdon, Cambridge and Bedfordshire Advertiser*, 23rd October, 1858, p.1.

"What, Ho! A Rat
Dead for a Ducat" – Hamlet.
Important to Farmers, Housekeepers, and Others.

Hartley's Lancashire Vermin Killer

Will be found on trial to be the most efficacious Preparation ever offered for the destruction of Rats, Mice. Black Beetles, and all other vermin. Rats will be found within a few feet of where the bait has been laid. Cats, Dogs , or other domestic animals will not touch it.

Sold in Packets, price 3d, 6d and 1s each.

PRODUCT
Harwood's Celebrated Vermin Killer

ORIGIN OF PRODUCT
H T Harwood, Pharmaceutical Chemist, 43 North Street, Taunton.

NOTES
Advert: *Chard and Ilminster News and Somerset, Dorset and Devon Advertiser*, 25th August, 1888, p.1.

PERFECT FREEDOM FROM VERMIN

DWELLING HOUSES, HOTELS, FARM BUILDINGS, GRANARIES, MILLS, STACKS, WAREHOUSES et cetera, SPEEDILY CLEARED OF RATS AND MICE BY *HARWOOD'S CELEBRATED VERMIN KILLER*.

NB. Admitted by those who use it to be the best preparation known for the destruction of Vermin of all kinds and cannot be excelled. Has been before the public for over twenty five years and never known to fail.

PRODUCT
Hewson's Vermin Killer

ORIGIN OF PRODUCT
John Hewson, Chemist, Mercer Row, Louth, Lincolnshire.

NOTES
Advert: *Louth and North Lincolnshire Advertiser,* 24th August, 1867, p.1.

Vermin Killer. At 3d, 6d and 1s per Packet.

PRODUCT
Heynes's Magic Vermin Killer

ORIGIN OF PRODUCT
W H Heynes, Chemist (by Examination), 28 High Street, Maidenhead.

NOTES
Advert: *Maidenhead Advertiser and Marlow Chronicle*, 8th March, 1876, p.4.

Heynes's Magic Vermin Killer.
For the extermination of Rats and Mice.
(Woodcut of rats eating and dying)

It's Effect is Sure.
Its Cost is Trifling.
It is Easily Applied.

Mice appear attracted to it as if by magic, eat it readily, tumble over, and **Die on the spot**.

Please observe that the above Woodcut is an exact facsimile of that on the wrapper in which *Heynes's Magic Vermin Killer* is sold. None other is genuine, and will disappoint in its results.

PRODUCT
Hill's Magic Vermin Killer

ORIGIN OF PRODUCT
Edward Hill, Wellington, Somerset.

NOTES
Advert: *York Herald*, 22nd September, 1874, p.2.

WONDERFUL.

A 3d Packet of *HILL'S MAGIC VERMIN KILLER* will destroy 50 MICE and 15 RATS. See Testimonials. Post free for 4, 7 or 12 stamps. AGENTS WANTED in every town, and will be supplied upon very liberal terms.

PRODUCT
Houlton's Vermin Killer

ORIGIN OF PRODUCT
James Houlton, Chemist (MPS by examination), 1 Market Place, Wetherby.

NOTES
Advert: *Tadcaster Post, and General Advertiser for Grimstone*, 3rd March, 1862, p.1.

PRODUCT
Hunter's Infallible Vermin Destroyer

NOTES
Advert: *Banner of Ulster*, 20th March, 1854, p.3.

RATS, MICE, COCKROACHES et cetera. WHAT NASTY THINGS THEY ARE! *HUNTER'S INFALLIBLE VERMIN DESTROYER* is recommended to parties troubled by them.

See text above *passim*

PRODUCT
Ingall's Vermin Killer

ORIGIN OF PRODUCT
J Ingall, Chemist, High Street, Ashford, Kent

NOTES
Advert: *Kentish Express*, 31st March, 1866, p.2

RATS! RATS! MICE! MICE!

Warehouses, Mills, Farm Buildings, Stacks, Granaries, et cetera speedily Cleared of Rats and Mice by

INGALL'S VERMIN KILLER

Mice eat it greedily, and die on the spot.

PRODUCT
Jones' Cheshire Vermin Killer

ORIGIN OF PRODUCT
Charles Jones, Chemist, Birkenhead.

NOTES
Advert: *Chester Courant and Advertiser for North Wales*, 21st February, 1855, p.5.

TO FARMERS, MILLERS & GAMEKEEPERS

The best and most simple method known for destroying Rats, Mice & Vermin in Covers et cetera.

Jones' Cheshire Vermin Killer; in pots with directions; 6d and 1s each.

PRODUCT
Kenny's Vermin Killer

ORIGIN OF PRODUCT
Thomas Kenny, Dispensing and Family Chemist, (Associate of the Pharmaceutical Society by Examination), Beverley Road, Stepney, Hull.

NOTES
Misuse
Inquest. Hannah Long, general servant, aged nineteen, found dead on the New Holland to Gainsborough train, at Kirton Lindsay station.

'Charles Frederick George said: I am a general practitioner and a Member of the Royal College of Surgeons. I received a parcel from Sergeant Baker containing two packets produced by last witness. One had been opened, one was still sealed. It was labelled "Kenny's Vermin Killer". Each packet contained a blue powder, and a quantity of strychnine; the unopened packet contained thirty grains of powder, the open one, which was partly used, only twelve grains. I could not say the exact proportions without an elaborate analysis. I have no doubt deceased died from taking part of the contents of the opened packet...I have not made a post mortem examination, but have seen the body of the deceased. She has the appearance of being pregnant.'

Source: *Lincolnshire Chronicle,* 25th August, 1882, p.7.

PRODUCT
LaPorte's Vermin Destroying Powder

ORIGIN OF PRODUCT
M La Porte, 31 Great James Street, Bedford Row, London.

NOTES
Advert: *Deal, Walmer and Sandwich Mercury*, 22nd August, 1868, p.4.

La Porte's Vermin Destroying Powders. Kills Rats and Mice. Sold in Packets 2s 6d and 5s. Sent post free anywhere.

PRODUCT
Levin's Magic Vermin Destroyer

NOTES
Advert: *Leicester Journal*, 19th December, 1862, p.5.

VERMIN! VERMIN!! VERMIN!!!

The great discovery of the age – *LEVIN'S MAGIC*

VERMIN DESTROYER. This celebrated preparation is certain death to black beetles, cockroaches, crickets, rats and mice. Thousands may be destroyed in one night, without danger to household pets. In consequence of immense demand Agents have been appointed in almost every town in the United Kingdom.

Insist on none but Levin's as there are many dangerous imitations.

PRODUCT
Linnell's Vermin Killer

ORIGIN OF PRODUCT
George Linnell, Chemist and Druggist, Market Place, Market Deeping, Lincolnshire.

NOTES
Misuse
Attempted suicide. 'On Saturday morning last John Mee, hawker and confectioner, of Deeping St James, attempted to commit suicide by taking a threepenny packet of *Linnell's Vermin Killer*, which he had himself purchased at Mr Linnell's shop at Market Deeping the same morning. On purchasing the poison he went home and spread it on some bread with lard, and

ate the greater portion of it. Mr. Deacon, surgeon, of Market Deeping, was immediately called in, and used every effort to save his life. He is now considered out of danger'.

Source: *Stamford Mercury*, 8th April, 1870, p.4.

PRODUCT
Lyon & Co's Vermin Killer

ORIGIN OF PRODUCT
H Lyon & Co, Corner of Petty Cury, Cambridge.

NOTES
Advert: *Cambridge Chronicle and Journal, Isle of Ely Herald and Huntingdonshire Gazette*, 14th June, 1856, p.5.

Persons troubled with Mice, Rats or Small birds, may at once destroy them, however numerous, by using *H Lyon and Co's Vermin Killer*. Sold in bottles at 6d, 1s and 1s and 9d each. To prevent disappointment H Lyon and Co caution their customers against buying of persons unknown to them. The genuine preparations being prepared with the greatest care by a chemical process by H Lyon and Co, Corner of Petty Cury, Cambridge.

NB The poison for rats is sold in a powder ready for mixing, with instructions.

PRODUCT
Mabson's Vermin Killer

ORIGIN OF PRODUCT
William Mabson, Pharmaceutical Chemist, Yarmouth.

NOTES
Advert: *Yarmouth Independent, North Norfolk and Eastern Counties Herald*, 4th January, 1862, p.8.

Mabson's Vermin Killer for destroying Rats, Mice, Beetles and Cockroaches. Mice particularly, eat it freely, AND DIE ON THE SPOT.
It is so CHEAP that hundreds may be destroyed for a few pence.

In private dwellings, it may be laid about safely, as you can take up in the morning what they do not eat.

No unpleasant smell is likely to arise as the Mice die chiefly within a short distance of the bait.

PRODUCT
Miller's Vermin and Insect Killer

ORIGIN OF PRODUCT
William Miller, Chemist, 137, Tithebarn Street, Liverpool.

NOTES
Advert: *Liverpool Albion*, 26th December, 1853, p.20.

Certain and speedy Death of Rats, Mice and Insects from Houses, Warehouses, Stacks, Farm Buildings, Vessels et cetera.

PRODUCT
Morris and Levin's Vermin Killer Powder

NOTES
Advert: *Leeds Mercury*, 21st May, 1859, p.3.

VERMIN! VERMIN! – IMPORTANT to FARMERS and Others. – "Oh, these rats, what shall I do to get rid of them?" Why, purchase a packet of MORRIS & *LEVIN'S VERMIN KILLING POWDER.*

PRODUCT
Patterson's Magic Vermin Killer

ORIGIN OF PRODUCT
George Patterson, Agricultural Chemist, Red Lion Square, Stamford.

NOTES
Advert: *Hull Advertiser*, 9th October, 1858, p.1

Magic Vermin Killer.

In Packets, price, 3d, 6d and 1s each.
(Vermin eat it readily, and die on the spot.)

PRODUCT
Priestley's Vermin Killer

NOTES
Advert: *The Halesworth Times and East Sussex Advertiser*, 8th December, 1857, p.1.

Farmers & Others.

BATS, MICE, and other VERMIN SPEEDILY DESTROYED BY *PRIESTLEY'S VERMIN KILLER*.

This Preparation is one of the most effective and speedy for the destruction of these Household and Farm-yard Pests that has ever been offered to public notice. The ingredients are of the most deadly character, but so compounded that it is eaten with the greatest avidity,—proving almost instant death. A small portion spread on thin pieces of bread, and placed in corn ricks, barns, or wherever the Vermin frequent, will be found eminently destructive. Those who have used it once will never use any other.

Sold in 6d. and Is Pots.

PRODUCT
Ramsden's Vermin Killer/Ramsden's Yorkshire Vermin Killer

NOTES
Advert: *Chester Courant and Advertiser for North Wales*, 11th May, 1859, p.1.

IMPORTANT TO AGRICULTURISTS, PRIVATE FAMILIES et cetera.

RAMSDEN'S VERMIN KILLER is the best and cheapest ever offered to the public, when used according to directions. Rats and Mice will it readily and die on the spot. Sold in packets at 3d., 6d., and 1s each.

PRODUCT
Reed's Vermin Killer

ORIGIN OF PRODUCT
William Rogers, Pharmaceutical Chemist, 34 High Street, Maidstone.

NOTES
Advert: *Maidstone Telegraph and West Kent Messenger*, 2nd January, 1863, p.1.
DEATH! DEATH!! DEATH!!!

TRY *REED'S VERMIN KILLER*, the most effectual destroyer of RATS and MICE ever discovered! Nearly 10,000 packets have been sold without a single advertisement!

NB. Ask for No 1 for Mice and Number 2 for Rats. Prepared exclusively and sold Wholesale and Retail by the proprietor, William Rogers.

PRODUCT
Sandford's Rat Poison

ORIGIN OF PRODUCT
Sandford and Son, Sandy, Bedfordshire.

NOTES
Advert: 28th March, 1883, *Melton Mowbray Mercury, and Oakham and Uppingham News*, 8th March, 1883, p.1.

RAT POISON. Any Poison will kill rats, the difficulty is to get them to eat it.

PRODUCT
Smith's Vermin Killer

ORIGIN OF PRODUCT
John Smith, chemist, Guildhall Street, Lincoln

NOTES
Misuse
Another Suicide in Lincoln

Inquest into death of Mrs Clarissa Sissons.

'Dr Lowe was called in at once, and pronounced life to

be quite extinct. On the deceased was found a packet labelled "Smith's Vermin Killer. Poison". This was empty. There was in her possession a piece of paper, on which was written in ink, "Mrs Sissons, Park cottages, No 1. My husband, I cannot live. Your wife, Clarissa Sissons". Verdict: suicide whilst temporarily insane'.

Source: *Lincolnshire Chronicle*, 19th January, 1892, p.3.

PRODUCT
Snartt's Vermin Destroyer

ORIGIN OF PRODUCT
Frederick Snartt, Chemist, 7 Red Lion Square, Stamford, Lincolnshire.

NOTES
Misuse
Inquest into death of George Gee, farmer of Deeping Fen, age sixty-three.

'Witness continued: these are the papers I took out of his trouser pocket. They were wrappers and labels which contained a quantity of *Snartt's Vermin Destroyer*, prepared by "Frederick Snartt, Chemist, Stamford" and labelled in bold type "Poison".

Source: *Lincolnshire Free Press*, 19th April, 1881, p.8.

PRODUCT
Spalding Chemical Vermin Killer

ORIGIN OF PRODUCT
Francis Milns, Chemist, Market Place, Spalding.

NOTES
Advert: *Stamford Mercury,* 6th July, 1849, p.1.

VERMIN! VERMIN!! VERMIN!!!

THE *SPALDING CHEMICAL VERMIN KILLER*

This Preparation is confidently recommended as the best that has hitherto been introduced for the destruction of Rats and Mice. Amongst other qualifications, it possesses the advantage of being so free from smell and taste that the Vermin greedily devour it, and it is so powerful that the smallest quantity destroys them on the spot, setting at rest any doubt about its efficacy.

The sale has been extensive at and around Spalding, and many testimonials of its efficacy have been received by the Proprietor. In pots at 6d and 1s each.

PRODUCT
Steiner's Rat Paste/ Steiner's Vermin Killer

ORIGIN OF PRODUCT
E Steiner, Henry Street, Limehouse, London.

NOTES
Listed by Alfred Allen.

Advert: *Shields Daily News*, 5th January, 1880, p.1.

Rats found Dead after using two 6d jars of *Steiner's Vermin Paste*. Sold by all Chemists. "Try it, it never fails".

Misuse
'Petty Sessions, Harleston. Henry Payne, baker of Pulham Market, charged with attempting suicide by taking poison…Mr John Nathaniel Legge Paulley, surgeon, Pulham Market, deposed that he was sent for to see Payne. He was nearly insensible. Witness judged from his appearance that the accused had taken some irritant. He seemed to be in pain and convulsed. Witness gave him an injection, and he was sick. The accused had certainly taken phosphorus, and witness knew that there was phosphorus in *Steiner's Vermin Killer*…sufficient in a bottle to kill a man'.

Source: *Star of the East*, 5th December, 1885, p.3.

PRODUCT
Thomas's Vermin Killer

ORIGIN OF PRODUCT
John Holiday Thomas, Market Place, Boston, Lincolnshire.

NOTES
Advert: *Stamford Mercury*, 21st September, 1855, p.1.

Thomas's Vermin Killer will speedily clear Houses, Stacks, Farm Buildings, and Warehouses of Rats and Mice, Beetles from Houses and Bakehouses, and Weasels, Magpies and Carrion Crows from Gentlemen's Preserves. Mice eat it readily and die on the spot. Rats more frequently die in their holes.

Prepared only by John Holiday Thomas, chemist, Boston, Lincolnshire.

PRODUCT
Thompson's Rat Paste and Vermin Killer

ORIGIN OF PRODUCT
Thomas Thompson, Chemist, Richmond, North Yorkshire.

NOTES
Advert: *Richmond and Ripon Chronicle*, 14th July, 1855, p.8.

PRODUCT
Thurston's Magic Vermin Killer

ORIGIN OF PRODUCT
Frederick Thurston, Chemist, Fressingfield, Sussex.

NOTES
Listed by Alfred Allen.

Misuse
The Charge of an Attempt to Poison a Child at Harleston.

Sarah Ann Snowling, domestic servant, accused of administering poison to her illegitimate son, George Snowling, aged fourteen months old, in a cake.
'Prisoner gave him threepence, and he went for the poison, which was supplied him by Mrs Thurston. There was something printed on the packet, though what it was he did not remember. [A small thin packet bearing a label was shown to witness by Superintendent Ward.] What was on the packet he

purchased was like that on the one produced, for he now distinctly recognised several of the words. The label on the packet produced by Superintendent Ward bore the following words:- "3d. Poison. 3d. *Thurston's Magic Vermin Killer*, effectually destroys rats, mice, beetles etc. Directions enclosed. Sold by all chemists. Manufactory, Long Melford, Suffolk'.

Source: *Norwich Mercury*, 14th February, 1874, p.7.

The Late Shocking Suicide by a Married Woman at Melford.

Inquest. 'Mr Frederick Thurston, pharmaceutical chemist, at Melford, produced his book, containing an entry dated June 6th, showing that he had sold a threepenny packet of vermin killer to the deceased's step-daughter, who signed her name. On the 19th October he sold another packet to Julia Simpson, who was then living as a servant with the deceased; not being able to read she made a mark. She told him when the purchase was made that she wanted some magic poison for killing mice'.

Source: *Bury and Suffolk Standard*, 3rd December, 1878, p.5.

PRODUCT
Twelvetrees's Mice and Rat Killer

ORIGIN OF PRODUCT
Harper Twelvetrees, the Works, Bromley by Bow, London.

NOTES
Advert: *Luton Times and Advertiser*, 4th December, 1858, p.4.

VERMIN! VERMIN! VERMIN!

They shall DIE and FOR EVER CEASE!!!

HARPER TWELVETREES' *INFALLIBLE AND IRRESISTABLE MICE AND RAT KILLER*, is the most delicious dainty ever prepared for Vermin!! It is not only so powerfully attractive as to decoy them from their holes, but is most certain and deadly in its effects. Mice cannot resist it!! They will follow it anywhere; eat it greedily, and die on the spot!!! You may clear them away by the score every night and morning. A Sixpenny Packet will kill 100 Mice and 50 Rats!!!

PRODUCT
Wise's Magic Vermin Killer

ORIGIN OF PRODUCT
J Wise APS, Dispensing Chemist, Market Square, St Neott's.

NOTES
Advert: *St Neott's Chronicle and Advertiser*, 20th March, 1880, p.1

MICE! RATS!! MICE!!!

Houses, Stacks, Farm Buildings, Warehouses, Mills et cetera, speedily cleared of Rats, Mice, Beetles, Cockroaches, et cetera, by

WISE'S MAGIC VERMIN KILLER

A Shilling Packet dresses a stack of 30 to 40 Quarters, and kills the Mice, frequently saving £5. IN PACKETS at 3d, 6d and 1s each.
MICE eat it readily and Die on the Spot. RATS more frequently Die in their Holes.

PRODUCT
Woodliffe's Vermin Killer

ORIGIN OF PRODUCT
Alfred Woodliffe, Chemist, 8 High Street, Bridlington.

NOTES
Advert: *Bridlington Free Press*, 17th February, 1872, p.4.

Woodliffe's Vermin Killer. Mice eat it greedily and die on the spot. 3d, 6d, 1/- and 2/- Packets.

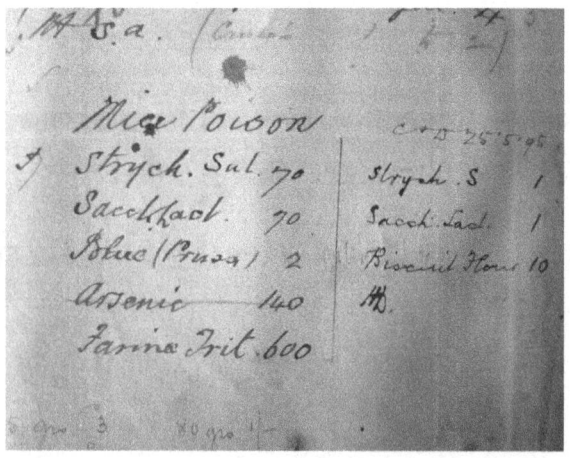

Chapter Two

'A person exceedingly dangerous': a short history of Elizabeth Vamplew, aged 13 years

Timeline

1848: Elizabeth Vamplew born in Grimoldby, near Louth, daughter of agricultural labourer, John Vamplew and his wife, Maria.

1st May, 1862: employed as nursemaid by Alvingham farmer, Edwin Taylor, and his wife, Mary.

1st July, 1862: Kate Mary Taylor, daughter of Edwin and Mary Taylor, aged eight weeks, taken ill, but recovers.

10th July, 1862: Kate Mary Taylor becomes very ill around 9 o'clock in the evening.

11th July, 1862: death of Kate Mary Taylor, at around 1.00 in the morning: suspicion falls on her nursemaid, 13 year old Elizabeth Vamplew.

: Elizabeth Vamplew taken into custody by Police Inspector William Roberts of Louth and charged with causing the death of an infant through the administration of poison.

12th July, 1862: inquest into the death of Kate Mary Taylor, in front of Dr Thomas Sharpley, coroner, at the Jolly Sailors Inn, Louth: adjourned.

16th July, 1862: resumed inquest at the Jolly Sailors Inn, Louth: adjourned a second time to await the evidence of Professor Alfred Swaine Taylor.

24th July, 1862: appears in front of the magistrates' bench at the Court House, Louth: committed for trial at the Lincoln Assizes.

25th July, 1862: delayed resumed inquest, at the Jolly Sailors Inn, Louth, found guilty of the wilful murder of Kate Mary Taylor by the coroner's jury.

26th July, 1862: received into Lincoln Castle prison, 2.30 in the afternoon, to await her trial at the Lincoln Assizes.

29th July, 1862: tried for the wilful murder of Kate Mary Taylor, at the Lincoln Assizes, in front of Chief Baron Frederick Pollock. Found guilty of manslaughter and sentenced to twelve years penal servitude.

1st September, 1862: removed from Lincoln Castle prison and received into Millbank prison, Surrey.
17th April, 1863: removed from Millbank prison and received into Parkhurst prison, Isle of Wight.
3rd July, 1866: removed from Parkhurst prison and received into Brixton prison, Lambeth.
9th March, 1867: released on licence from Brixton prison on medical grounds.
15th December,1867: buried at Grimoldby, aged 18 years.

The popular press was spoilt for choice when it came to constructing a sensational headline with which to engage its readers in the story of Elizabeth Vamplew.

The *Lincolnshire Chronicle* and the *Stamford Mercury* both focused upon the appalling death of an infant in Alvingham, near Louth, with the headline, 'Child Poisoning'; on the other hand, the *Grantham Journal* highlighted a shocking betrayal of domestic trust with the words, 'Murder of a Child by its Nurse'.

Whilst the death of an infant in suspicious circumstances was depressingly commonplace at the time, the alleged perpetrator of the crime being only thirteen years of age was not. The journalistic shock value of such an unusual occurrence was not lost on some newspapers, especially outside Lincolnshire, which drew attention to the story with the headline, 'Murder by a Child'. However, in terms of gothic sensationalism, nothing surpassed the *Edinburgh Evening Courant* and Selkirk's *Southern Reporter*, which began their account of Elizabeth Vamplew's subsequent trial and conviction with the headline, 'A Juvenile Fiend'.

The more restrained newspaper headlines used either the adjective 'strange' or 'extraordinary' to describe the alleged murder of the eight week old child. These claims were true enough, but not quite in the way the newspapers understood them.

INQUEST INTO THE DEATH OF KATE MARY TAYLOR, AGED EIGHT WEEKS, IN FRONT OF DR THOMAS SHARPLEY, CORONER, 12TH JULY, 1862, AT THE JOLLY SAILORS INN, LOUTH

The inquest into the death of Kate Mary Taylor turned out to be a somewhat protracted and convoluted business in that it was twice adjourned by the coroner before the jury was in a position to pronounce its verdict on the circumstances presented to it.

The fullest report of the beginning of the extended process was published in the *Lincolnshire Chronicle*, on 18th July, although the story was also covered by the *Stamford Mercury*, on the same day, and less usefully by the *Grantham Journal*, a day later.

The opening of the report on the inquest was

sober in tone, outlining the known facts of the case relating to the infant daughter of Alvingham farmer, Edwin Taylor, whose death appeared to have been caused by the administration of poison.

The first witness to depose was the father of the dead child, who stated that his daughter had been very ill two weeks prior to the inquest and had presented 'appearances of a suspicious nature'. No details were given of the symptoms which had caused such alarm, but the child had recovered and no further notice had been taken.

On the Thursday evening of the 10th July, Kate Mary Taylor was left 'for a few minutes' in the hands of the young nursemaid, Elizabeth Vamplew, and shortly afterwards, the infant began to cry. In response, Mary Taylor, the mother, investigated the problem, at which point the infant began 'shrieking fearfully' and was 'in great agony': Kate Mary Taylor died at around 1 o'clock in the morning.

During the course of that day, Edwin Taylor said, his other servant girl told him that Elizabeth Vamplew had confessed to her that she had given the child mouse poison. In response, he took the young girl to Louth, presumably to meet the coroner or the police, or both, and on the journey, Elizabeth Vamplew told her master that she had indeed poisoned the infant, not with mouse poison, but with white mercury, and that she had obtained the poison from her mother without her knowledge. It was a strange fine distinction by the suspected murderer which made little difference in terms of legalities, but it was one with which she persisted.

The statement made by Edwin Taylor, not surprisingly, was confirmed as being absolutely true by Betsy Clarke, the servant girl who had reported the alleged confession of Elizabeth Vamplew.

The next deposition, from Mary Wright, the wife of the Grimoldby shopkeeper, John Wright, was a crucial one. She confirmed that she had sold a packet of *Battle's Vermin Killer*, the most popular solution to domestic problems with mice, to Elizabeth Vamplew.

The oddness of Elizabeth Vamplew claiming that she had used white mercury to kill the baby, rather than *Battle's Vermin Killer*, was further complicated by the deposition of Maria Vamplew, her mother, who assured the coroner's court that she hadn't had any white mercury in the house since May Day.

The deposition of the Louth surgeon, John B Wroe, who had carried out a post mortem on Kate Mary Taylor, was cautious and therefore a qualified one. On examining the body, he had found internal symptoms 'such as would lead him to believe that some irritant poison had been introduced into the stomach'. The analysis confirmed that a felony had probably been committed, but was not helpful in terms of the clarifying the exact nature of the poison which had been administered to kill the child.

At this point, the inquest was adjourned until the evening of the following Wednesday.

RESUMED INQUEST INTO THE DEATH OF KATE MARY TAYLOR, AGED EIGHT WEEKS, IN FRONT OF DR THOMAS SHARPLEY, CORONER, 16TH JULY, 1862, AT THE JOLLY SAILORS INN, LOUTH

If the initial inquest, as reported by the *Lincolnshire Chronicle*, appeared to be somewhat pedestrian, its continuation, in part, produced interesting new details of the case which were more helpful, at least in terms of understanding the circumstantial evidence which pointed to Elizabeth Vamplew's involvement in the death of an infant.

The opening of the resumed inquest, however, was not very promising, in that Betsy Clarke was recalled 'without any fresh facts being elicited', and Mary Taylor, the mother of the unfortunate infant, provided evidence which 'entirely corroborated that of her husband'. The newspaper assured the reader that her deposition had been more explicit than her husband's in terms of describing the symptoms of the child's distressing condition and it had enabled the coroner and the jury 'to form a more correct opinion of the cause of death', but it did not elaborate.

The testimony of William Mitchell, the father of Mary Taylor, was more helpful and appeared to be decisive in establishing a motive, albeit a curious one, for the administration of poison to his granddaughter by young Elizabeth Vamplew.

William Mitchell had been taking tea at his daughter's house on the day of the death of Kate Mary Taylor when Betsy Clarke entered the room and told him that the nurse girl Vamplew had admitted giving the child mouse poison. Going upstairs, he found her crying and he asked her directly if she had given the baby anything, to which she replied that she had. Enquiring why she had done so, she said that it was because she was tired of 'hugging it about'. Whilst being taken away to Louth, she had also admitted that she had inserted poison powder into the baby's mouth with her finger and that she had obtained it from her mother's desk.

Clearly requiring much more precise information relating to the medical aspects of the case, Dr Sharpley once again adjourned the inquest to await the report of Professor Swaine Taylor, to whom the stomach and intestines of Kate Mary had been sent that day for analysis in London.

The *Lincolnshire Chronicle* report ended at this point as the coroner had not fixed a date for the resumption of the inquest.

The account of the inquest published in the *Stamford Mercury*, described as 'the substance of the evidence adduced', broadly duplicated the report found in the *Lincolnshire Chronicle*, although it is clear that the writer was reporting on the initial inquest only. The report ended by recording that the inquest had been adjourned until the following Wednesday, and then a second time *sine die*, in order to take account of the report of Professor Swaine Taylor.

However, the Stamford newspaper did include material not mentioned in the *Lincolnshire Chronicle* and which in some respects appeared to contradict it.

According to the *Stamford Mercury*, the baby was left in the charge of Elizabeth Vamplew, and that Mr and Mrs Taylor had retired to bed for the night, leaving her with the child 'for a short time.' On hearing her daughter crying, Mrs Taylor went downstairs and took it back into her chamber, where it 'shrieked fearfully and was in awful agony', until dying at 1 o'clock in the morning. At this point, the account had only departed marginally from that found in the Lincoln newspaper.

What followed was considerably different, however, in that it reported that Mr Taylor, suspecting that all was not well, had travelled to Louth to consult the coroner about the death of his baby daughter, but unfortunately, he was not at home. In the evening, whilst he was preparing to go to Louth once again, he was interrupted by Betsy Clarke who informed him that Elizabeth Vamplew had confessed to the killing. As a result, he took Elizabeth Vamplew in his gig to Louth and on the journey there she admitted to poisoning the child with white mercury, but denied the use of mouse powder.

The report on the post mortem by Mr Wroe was less bland than in the version published in the Lincoln newspaper, noting that he had found the chin and the lips of the dead child discoloured, and the membranes of the stomach covered with red streaks and patches. These observations and 'other facts' led him to suppose that irritant poison had entered the stomach of the child.

The report found in the *Grantham Journal* the next day was clearly taken from the *Stamford Mercury*, whose account it duplicates almost verbatim.

SECOND RESUMED INQUEST INTO THE DEATH OF KATE MARY TAYLOR, AGED EIGHT WEEKS, IN FRONT OF DR THOMAS SHARPLEY, CORONER, 25th JULY, 1862, AT THE JOLLY SAILORS INN, LOUTH

Because the second resumption of the inquest had no fixed date, the newspapers trying to track the case were somewhat disadvantaged in terms of a smooth continuity of reporting.

The *Lincolnshire Chronicle*, like the *Stamford Mercury*, was published on a Friday, and its report of the 25th July, seemed to have been seriously hampered by uncertainties surrounding the formal resumption of the inquest caused by the delayed report of Professor Swaine Taylor.

Unable to produce an account of the second resumption of the inquest, the *Lincolnshire Chronicle* began with a short notice of the appearance of Elizabeth Vamplew in front of the county magistrates at the Louth Court House on the previous Thursday: the Bench had consisted of Mr William Henry Smyth, Lord Frederick Beauclerk and Mr Cornelius Parker.

Unfortunately, there is a sense that the reporter was both flustered and unclear about the circumstances relating to the developing story he was supposed to be recounting, which resulted in a masterpiece of journalistic confusion.

The reminder to the reader that details of the case had been reported the previous week seemed like a convenient escape clause, rather than a helpful recap, as was the vague assurance that the evidence against the prisoner, coupled with the statements made by her, appeared to be 'very strong'. That the reporter had renamed the child poisoner as Mary Vamplew did not inspire confidence in a firm grasp of the facts.

The account of the appearance of Elizabeth Vamplew in front of the magistrates which consisted merely of a passing mention of Betsy Clarke, whose evidence was 'substantially the same as on the previous Saturday', was a further indication of a desperate attempt to create a story built on flimsy knowledge. His reference to the previous deposition of Betsy Clarke at the initial inquest, as reported by the *Lincolnshire Chronicle* of 18th July, was totally unhelpful. The words of the domestic servant were never recorded, only generalised into a deposition which, it was claimed, did not disagree with that of her master; even if the reader had remembered that Betsy Clarke had been recalled to the witness stand at the first resumed inquest on the following Wednesday, he would have been left disappointed, in that the newspaper reported that nothing new had been added. There is a sense that in his muddle, the reporter was transposing information from the first resumed inquest into a vague account of the proceedings in the Louth magistrates' court, which in itself may have been a desperate partial invention.

The confusions continued when the reporter tried to explain the uncertainties surrounding the expected report from Professor Swaine Taylor, upon which a good deal depended in terms of an accurate analysis of the cause of Kate Mary Taylor's death. It is clear from the ambiguous and perplexing chronology that the reporter thought the evidence of the distinguished toxicologist had been due on either

Saturday the 12th July, which was impossible, or on the following Saturday, the 19th July, which was probable, in that the bottles containing the relevant body parts, it later transpired, had reached London on Thursday 17th July. However, the reporter produced further difficulties by telling his readers that Inspector Roberts of the Louth police had been soon expected to be back from London, 'with evidence as to the analysis of the stomach of the deceased infant by Professor Taylor'. He seemed to be naively unaware of the fixed protocols and procedures of a coroner's inquest when involving an expert medical witness such as Alfred Swaine Taylor delivering vital forensic evidence. In addition, the possibility that the eminent toxicologist would have entrusted his report to be presented in court by a Louth police officer was risible.

To some extent, the reporter managed to dig himself out of the bewildering hole he had dropped himself into by informing the reader that Elizabeth Vamplew was 'again brought before the magistrates, on Saturday, as the scientific evidence was wanting' and that she was 'again remanded until Tuesday'.

The final sentence brought a semblance of closure to the journalistic fiasco by stating that the inquest had not resumed 'in consequence of no communication having been received from Professor Taylor'.

The confusions of the *Lincolnshire Chronicle*, to some extent, were resolved the next day by the *Louth and North Lincolnshire Advertiser*, which seemed to have a more secure understanding of events, having had a day longer to discover and digest reliable information.

There was no extended account of the second resumed inquest, which it turned out had only taken place on the night of Friday, 25th July: but in an appended paragraph, it reported that the coroner's court had eventually heard the report of Professor Swaine Taylor and that the jury had unanimously returned a verdict of Guilty against Elizabeth Vamplew.

Unusually, the formal examination of the prisoner in front of the magistrates had taken place on the afternoon of Friday, 25th July, at 2.15, well before the verdict of the coroner's court had been reached.

Unsurprisingly, perhaps, the composition of the Bench reported in the *Louth and North Lincolnshire Advertiser* was not exactly the same as that found in the muddled report published in the *Lincolnshire Chronicle*: it consisted of the Reverend W Smyth, Mr William Henry Smyth (Chairman), Mr Henry Pye and Mr Cornelius Parker.

The main focus of the hearing was the report of Professor Swaine Taylor, but he was preceded by Edwin Taylor, the father of the alleged victim of poison.

The deposition of Edwin Taylor differed considerably from that heard previously in that it explained in some detail the first illness of his daughter which he had only mentioned briefly at the coroner's inquest. The latest account not only provided additional information concerning the symptoms of the mystery illness of the infant, but also implicated Elizabeth Vamplew as part of the embellished narrative.

According to Mr Taylor, the baby had first showed signs of illness in its sleep, but neither he nor his wife could work out what was wrong. Between 10 o'clock in the morning and 4 o'clock in the afternoon his daughter suffered from convulsions, and also shrieked and whined when she occasionally woke from her disturbed sleep. During the course of these distressing occurrences, Elizabeth Vamplew 'was nursing it all the time'. Edwin Taylor insisted that the child had enjoyed previous good health and 'had never been attacked in this way before'; he also insisted, in a somewhat garbled re-hash of the final hours of Kate Mary two weeks later, that she was comfortably asleep on the knee of Elizabeth Vamplew when he left her.

It is perhaps odd that on neither of these occasions did Edwin Taylor seek the advice and support of a doctor.

The apparently elusive Professor Taylor presented his report to the Bench, noting that he had received two well-sealed glass bottles and a packet of

Battle's Vermin Killer, on Thursday, 17th July, from Superintendent Roberts. The glass bottles had contained the stomach and viscera of an infant child; the packet of *Battle's Vermin Killer* contained three-quarters of a grain of strychnine.

In the opinion of the expert toxicologist, there was no poison in the stomach and intestines of the infant, although the mucous liquid found on the stomach, upon close analysis, showed traces of strychnine. Further, there was no evidence of disease in the stomach or the viscera, which might have accounted for death.

Professor Taylor concluded that the cause of death was strychnine poison, noting that only a quarter of the powder found in a packet of *Battle's Vermin Killer* would be needed to kill even a grown man.

The analysis was decisive: Mr William Henry Smyth, after consulting with the rest of the Bench, committed Elizabeth Vamplew to the next session of the Lincoln Assizes, to be tried for wilful murder.

The pre-trial processing of Elizabeth Vamplew was clinically efficient. She was received into Lincoln Castle prison on the afternoon of Saturday 26th July, at 2.30, along with two debtors, Robert Bell and Robert Ranshaw. On account of her age, James Foster, the Prison Governor, 'ordered it advisable to place her in association with another prisoner for trial', according to his *Journal* for that day.

The *Journal* of the Prison Matron for the same day noted that the allocated prisoner in question was Hannah Stubley, 'by order of the surgeon'.

The existence of Elizabeth Vamplew was recorded in the *Journal* of Henry Richter, the Prison Chaplain, on Sunday, 27th July, but without comment. Later encounters with her were minimal, consisting of a visit on the day after her conviction and final spiritual advice on the Sunday before she was removed to Millbank prison, on the 1st September.

TRIAL OF ELIZABETH VAMPLEW, IN FRONT OF CHIEF BARON FREDERICK POLLOCK, 29TH JULY, 1862, AT THE LINCOLN ASSIZES

On Monday, 28th July, at 1.30, the prisoner was examined by the Prison Surgeon, Ralph Howett, along with two other prisoners, to ensure that she was fit to stand trial the next day.

The earliest reporting of the trial of Elizabeth Vamplew was published on Wednesday, 30th July, in the London based newspaper, *The Sun*, as part of its report on the business of the Midland Circuit. Large parts of it were duplicated in the *Sheffield Independent* and the *Leeds Mercury* the following day.

Whilst the account found in the London newspaper was not contradicted in its essentials by the two later Lincolnshire newspaper reports, it does provide occasional supplementary details which give an additional clarity to some of the events in question. Unfortunately, it also includes some indisputable factual errors, such as the time of death of the Kate Mary Taylor.

The report on the business of the Assize published in the *Lincolnshire Chronicle* on Friday, 1st August, began as usual with local pride in the civic pomp and ceremony of the occasion, including the customary presentation of a pair of handsomely embroidered white gloves to the Crown Court judge by the City Sherriff, Mr Reuben Trotter.

At 2 o'clock on Saturday, 26th July, along with Lord Chief Justice William Earle, Lord Chief Baron Frederick Pollock had arrived in the city by train from Nottingham. They had been met by the High Sherriff, Mr T J Dixon, his Chaplain, the Reverend G Garfit, the Under-Sherriff and various other officials, before being transported to County Hall in the splendour of the High Sherriff's carriage. There, the Lord Chief Baron had opened the Commission for the County, before being taken to the Sessions House to open the Commission for the City.

Civic pleasantries and religious duties behind him, Chief Baron Pollock took his seat at the Crown Court on Monday, 28th July, at 11 o'clock precisely and following the usual preliminaries, the Grand Jury was sworn in. It was a formidable list of both experience and influence:

> Honourable Alexander Leslie Melville (Foreman)
> Honourable Charles Henry John Anderson
> Henry Hickman Bacon
> Thomas Chaplin
> Sir Montague John Cholmeley, MP
> Thomas G Corbett
> Richard Ellison
> John Lewis Ffytche
> Honourable Robert North Collie Hamilton
> George Fieschi Heneage
> William Hutton
> George Knowles Jarvis
> Charles Thomas James Moore
> Charles Massingberd-Mundy
> George Nevile
> George Hussey Packe
> William Parker
> Wilkinson Peacock
> John Reeve
> William Henry Smyth
> Sir John Trollope
> William Earle Welby
> Anthony Willson

The opening address by Judge Pollock to the Grand Jury was a mixed bag of compliment and complaint. On the one hand, the Calendar contained a larger number of prisoners than was usual 'in this generally peaceable county'; on the other, whilst the city of Lincoln was without a single prisoner, the Calendar did contain 'a large number of charges for a variety of heinous offences' committed elsewhere in Lincolnshire.

A late addition to the Calendar was the case of a young girl employed by a farming family in Alvingham who had been charged with murder. On the evidence of the depositions which the Chief Baron had read, it appeared that an infant had been poisoned and that 'whatever might be said in favour of the prisoner, without doubt the circumstances were such as to justify the Grand Jury returning a true bill.'

The gentlemen of the Grand Jury did not disappoint and the trial of Elizabeth Vamplew took place on Tuesday, 29th July, preceded by two cases of concealment of a birth. In both cases, the women accused, both domestic servants, were found Not Guilty and acquitted; Elizabeth Vamplew, unsurprisingly, was not so lucky.

The *Lincolnshire Chronicle* published its comprehensive report on the trial, beginning with a description of 'a delicate looking girl' seemingly lost in the dock. When asked to make her plea, she 'scarcely seemed aware of the position in which she was placed' and pleaded Guilty. However, she was subsequently advised to change her plea to Not Guilty.

The Counsel for the Prosecution consisted of Mr John B Sargeaunt and Mr Lewis Cave, whilst the case for the Defence was undertaken, at the request of the judge, by Mr Edward Chandos Leigh.

Mr Sargeaunt opened proceedings by earnestly requesting the jury to forget anything they had read in the newspapers or rumours which they might have heard outside the courtroom: their attention should be focused entirely upon the words of the witnesses only in reaching a verdict. After reminding the jury of the facts of the case, he distilled the issues down to two simple questions: was the infant poisoned by strychnine and if so, by whom was it administered?

Before the first witness was called, the learned counsel also helpfully reminded the jury that the prisoner in the dock was only thirteen and a half years old, and therefore they should be mindful of the question of criminal responsibility: in a legal sense, was Elizabeth Vamplew fully aware that she was acting wrongly when administering poison?

Before sitting down, Mr Sargeaunt expressed an unwavering confidence in the judgment of the gentlemen of the jury.

The various testimonies of Edwin Taylor, the father of the dead infant, as reported in the local newspapers, had been distinguished by the increasing amount of circumstantial detail which he provided. More precisely, they were distinguished by the increasing amount of evidence which defined the character and alleged actions of Elizabeth Vamplew.

He began his deposition by telling the court that the prisoner had been in his employment as a nursemaid since May Day and that he had three children. According to the earlier report in *The Sun*, Elizabeth Vamplew had entered the service of the Taylor household 'without a character', which presumably meant without any kind of formal endorsement concerning her suitability to work as a nursemaid. However, this does not seem to have been mentioned by Mr Taylor in any of his depositions.

The starting date of her employment may have seemed a trivial piece of domestic contextual information only, but an alert juryman might have viewed it as more than that in the light of Maria Vamplew's claim at the inquest that she had not had any white mercury in her house since May Day.

The testimony of Edwin Taylor heard in front of the Louth magistrates concentrated a good deal on the illness of his daughter two weeks before her death. In his latest account of events, he focused more upon the tragic events of Thursday 10th and Friday 11th July.

He recalled that on the Thursday Elizabeth

Vamplew had been given permission to attend the school feast at Grimoldby, her home village, around five miles away. He did not go into any detail about the school feast, but it was almost certainly the celebration by the Grimoldby Free Methodists of the fifth anniversary of their Sunday School, which according to the *Louth and North Lincolnshire Advertiser*, 'provided a bountiful supply of plum cake and tea for the children and adults'.

Elizabeth Vamplew returned to her place of employment about 9 o'clock that evening and after she had changed into her work clothes Mrs Taylor put her in charge of her baby daughter. Shortly afterwards, Mr Taylor followed his wife upstairs to bed, but within a few minutes, they heard the baby crying, and so Mrs Taylor went down and brought her infant daughter into the bedroom.

The child continued to cry a little and so after putting out the light, Mrs Taylor tried to breast feed it, but without much success: almost immediately the child began to scream. Thinking that she had been accidentally pricked by a pin, Mrs Taylor told her husband to provide a light in order to investigate the matter, but without being able to find a pin. On lighting the candle, Mr Taylor instead had discovered the horrific sight of the child frothing at the mouth and evidently in great agony; in addition, her stiff limbs were twitching and she was sweating profusely.

The scene for Mrs Taylor in particular was distressing, and after handing the baby over to her husband, she fainted.

The baby endured its appalling agonies until around 1 o'clock in the morning, when she died.

According to Mr Taylor, he saw Elizabeth Vamplew about 5 o'clock that morning and asked her if she had given Kate Mary any food to eat on the previous night. Given the time frame of only a few minutes between her having taken the baby, putting it on her knee and it starting to cry, it seemed a rather glib question. However, a supplementary question, though stranger still, was perhaps more to the point: had she put 'any of that stuff off your head into its mouth'? What he meant precisely by 'that stuff' was not explained in the report, but the nursemaid denied giving the baby either food or 'stuff'.

After he went upstairs, he heard Elizabeth Vamplew go into her own bedroom, unlock her box and then lock it up again. Mrs Taylor questioned her as to why she had gone upstairs to her room and was told that it was to retrieve a dirty apron.

Mr Taylor's account of the unfolding events of that day suggests increasing suspicion and an urgent search for certainties. Moving from his gentle, early morning coaxing of Elizabeth Vamplew, he became more direct and confrontational in his questioning. Whilst in the kitchen, he asked her about the contents of a bottle which he knew she kept in her box, to which she replied that it was 'toothache stuff her mother had sent her'. On being challenged to show him the bottle, the nursemaid went to a desk in the kitchen and produced the bottle in question. Mr Taylor asserted that the bottle was his, not hers, but she insisted that 'it was the bottle she had the stuff in'.

If Edwin Taylor's recollection was accurate, he seems at this point to have given up on trying to get some clarity on the bottle and its contents, falling back on the more secure ground of threatening to call for an inquest in order to resolve the mystery of his daughter's death.

If the master of the house was expecting his servant to crumble at the possibility of a public enquiry into the death of Kate Mary Taylor and own up to being involved in it, he was to be disappointed. The response of the thirteen-year old Elizabeth Vamplew was not the hoped for trembling admission of responsibility, but rather an astonishing confidential sharing of personal experience. According to a well-informed and perhaps slightly piqued Elizabeth Vamplew, her mother's child had died in exactly the same way as his daughter in the previous year, as had the baby of Mrs Brumby, but no inquest was ever held on either of them.

The two infant deaths were not an invention: her sister, Charlotte Vamplew, aged about eight months, was buried on the 7th April, 1861, coincidentally the day of the Census, in which she was not therefore recorded; whilst a William Ingleby Bromby, the son of William and Mary Bromby, residents of Manby Hall, was interred on the 1st July, 1861, and was recorded as being 0 years old in the *Burial Register* of the nearby village of Manby.

The precision of the local knowledge of Elizabeth Vamplew on such matters may have surprised Edwin Taylor; what may have surprised him even more, although he did not say so in his testimony, was the observation made by his domestic servant that whilst Mrs Bromby's baby had died in the same way as Mr Taylor's daughter, it had taken an hour and a quarter to die.

This matter of fact imparting of knowledge about infants enduring an unpleasant death and a comparative analysis of the time taken to die did not seem to elicit any comment in court, although it may have provided some later commentators on the case with speculative evidence of multiple murders carried out by the young girl.

Edwin Taylor concluded his appearance on the witness stand by confirming that he went to see the coroner after eating his dinner.

Mrs Taylor, called by Mr Sargeaunt, once again dutifully confirmed the truth of what her husband had told the court. In response to a question from the Counsel for the Defence, she said that it was the prisoner's duty to attend to the other children in the house. Unfortunately for Mr Chandos Leigh, Mary Taylor also told the court that she had not been satisfied with the domestic work of Elizabeth Vamplew and even more damning, she considered her to be 'a deceitful girl'. Mrs Taylor was also questioned directly by the Chief Baron concerning the previous illness of her daughter. She informed the court that Kate Mary was ailing about a month before her death – which was a different time scale to that previously heard – and that in response to her daughter's illness she had sent for a woman 'who understood children'. In the opinion of the woman who understood children, the illness of the baby was down to it having had some 'sleepy stuff'. The nature of the substance seems to have remained as imprecise and vague as the identity of the woman herself.

Betsy Clarke, the other domestic servant working in the Taylor household, had appeared at the three inquests and at the magistrates' court. Whilst she was perhaps the most significant witness for the case against Elizabeth Vamplew, what she deposed was never reported verbatim in the newspapers. It was merely recorded in terms of consistency with what had been said by Edwin Taylor or noted as being little different to her previous deposition. The incriminating words of Betsy Clarke concerning the confession of Elizabeth Vamplew were heard in court, but they were mediated by Edwin Taylor and his father-in-law, William Mitchell, to whom they were allegedly addressed on Friday, 11th July.

At the trial, however, the *Lincolnshire Chronicle* was able to report directly the further damning revelations concerning her conversations with the prisoner, as Betsy Clarke responded to the questions of Mr Cave.

She recalled the prisoner going to the school feast at Grimoldby, returning home and then getting into bed with her. After a short time, she was called to get some warm water for the baby. The report in *The Sun*, confirmed the reason for this request by way of noting that Mary Taylor had placed her baby in warm water in response to its convulsions.

Whilst Betsy Clarke was attending to this unwelcome domestic duty, Elizabeth Vamplew had also got out of bed and had taken a look round the door into her mistress's chamber.

In what reads like a telescoping of events and conversations, Betsy Clarke had asked Elizabeth Vamplew to get up, but she had refused on account of her being of no use if she did so, followed by a return to bed and announcing that the baby was dead. The response to the news was somewhat underwhelmed: 'Oh is it?' was the alleged minimal response from Elizabeth Vamplew.

During the morning, she told her that the master had decided to report the unexplained death in order to seek the judgement of a coroner's jury. In response to this development, she had allegedly asked Betsy Clarke, 'Will they know whether it is poisoned or not?' Betsy Clarke had assured her that they would, but Elizabeth Vamplew remained sceptical about the competence of a jury consisting of local farmers and tradesmen: 'How can they know, they are only men like my master.'

Crucially, Betsy Clarke was clear that she had never mentioned the subject of poisoning before the conversation took place.

William Mitchell, the father of Mary Taylor, by his own account at the resumed inquest, had been an important witness to the events and conversations of Friday, 11th July: Betsy Clarke had informed him of the confession of Elizabeth Vamplew as to having used mouse poison to kill the infant and he had therefore gone upstairs to talk to her about the matter. He had discovered a much distressed girl who was crying, who admitted to the crime and who also explained her reason for committing it.

In his latest appearance in a courtroom, William Mitchell gave a modified version of his earlier reported deposition, and at the same time, added significantly to it. His account made no mention of Betsy Clarke having spoken to him whilst eating tea with the family:

his latest version was less of a deliberate interrogation of Elizabeth Vamplew than a concerned conversation after having heard her crying in her bedroom. He had asked her why she was crying, to which the young girl said that she didn't know. William Mitchell then put the question directly to Elizabeth Vamplew: 'Surely you have not given the child anything?' The sudden bluntness of the question, as reported by the *Lincolnshire Chronicle,* was perhaps more apparent than real: the account of Mr Mitchell's deposition in *The Sun*, reported that his question was preceded by the tearful Elizabeth Vamplew asking him if she would be sent to prison.

The nursemaid had then admitted to William Mitchell that she had administered poison to the child. In addition to the confession, but certainly not mentioned in his earlier deposition, Elizabeth Vamplew also told him that 'she did not think the poison would kill it so soon'. It was an alleged remark which recalled the similar unhealthy interest in how long poison took to kill a baby, deposed by Edwin Taylor.

Seemingly keen to discover further details of the crime, William Taylor asked Elizabeth Vamplew if the poison was in a liquid or powder form, to which she replied that it was in powder form. His interview with the young girl ended with her enigmatic explanation of her motive for poisoning the child, heard previously at the resumed inquest.

The only question from Mr Chandos Leigh to William Mitchell seemed an innocuous one concerning his reasons for questioning Elizabeth Vamplew. His response was that Betsy Clarke had revealed that she had confessed to poisoning the child. The theme of the high pressure questioning of a young girl was one to which the Counsel for the Defence would later return in his closing remarks.

Mary Wright, the wife of Grimoldby grocer and draper, John Wright, under examination remembered Elizabeth Vamplew coming into the shop between 2 and 3 o'clock on the school feast day. She had asked to buy a penny doll and had then asked if Mrs Wright had any mouse poison? She said that she had, went to her drawer and brought out a packet of *Battle's Vermin Killer*. Mrs Wright enquired who had sent her to buy the poison and she was told that it was her mistress who had sent her. Pressing the point, she asked if she had been unable to buy any poison nearer to the Taylor house, in Cockerington, to which she replied that she couldn't. Elizabeth Vamplew departed with her purchases and was warned by Mrs Wright to take good care of the packet of *Battle's Vermin Killer*, as it contained poison.

There is a strong sense, in comparison with her earlier testimony at the initial inquest, that Mrs Wright was keen to provide details which the court might find helpful, and at the same time, make it abundantly clear that she had acted with great caution and discretion when selling poison to a girl of thirteen.

Unfortunately for Mary Wright, Judge Frederick Pollock was less impressed with her than she was with herself. His tart observation in response to the assurance that she had told the young girl to take care of the deadly packet was to suggest that she should have taken care of it herself by not having sold it to her.

Perhaps in a feeble attempt to rescue her tattered reputation for being a responsible citizen, Mary Wright told the court that she had four packets of *Battle's Vermin Killer* in the house on the 11th and 12th July, and had dutifully handed over two of them to policemen. She also revealed that she knew Elizabeth Vamplew, whose father was a labouring man, and that the girl had spent five weeks in her service. Unfortunately, Mrs Wright did not provide any information concerning the circumstances of the prisoner having worked for her and for only a short time.

Inspector William Roberts of Louth police confirmed that he had taken Elizabeth Vamplew into custody and had charged her with causing the death of an infant by administering poison. Once again, the prisoner had protested, not her innocence, but the means by which she murdered the infant: 'It's a misunderstanding: it was white mercury I gave the child; I got it from my mother's drawer when she was out'. On the evening of the 11th July, he had searched through the box of Elizabeth Vamplew, but had found neither white mercury nor *Battle's Vermin Killer*.

The inspector deposed that he had carried out his professional duties by taking the body of the dead child to Mr Wroe, surgeon of Louth, for examination, and had also taken a sealed packet to London for Professor Taylor's examination.

John Wroe confirmed that he had conducted an examination of the body of Kate Mary Taylor and that he had found the heart, lungs and heart perfectly healthy. He had sealed the stomach in one glass and the intestines in another, and had then handed them over to Inspector Roberts for delivery to London.

The final witness, almost inevitably, was Professor Alfred Swaine Taylor of Guy's Hospital, who went through the process of his examination in meticulous detail.

The professor confirmed that he had received a paper parcel and a packet of *Battle's Vermin Killer* in London on the 17th July: one parcel contained the stomach of the deceased child and the second parcel the intestines. On examining the stomach and intestines minutely he had found them perfectly healthy. Re-examining them separately, he had discovered a small quantity of strychnine in the stomach, but none in the intestines. The quantity of strychnine was a fraction of a grain: having found evidence of the poison in the stomach, it was natural to suppose that a part of it had been absorbed into the blood stream and had caused death.

An examination of the packet of *Battle's Vermin Killer* revealed the presence of three-quarters of a grain of strychnine. In his experience, the quantity of strychnine found in *Battle's Vermin Killer* varied from a single grain to half a grain. The remaining contents consisted of flour, starch and a small quantity of Prussian Blue to give it colour: a small quantity of the powder would be sufficient to destroy the life of a ten week old child. In addition to the forensic evidence, the symptoms of twitching and jumping pointed to the irresistible conclusion that Kate Mary Taylor had died from the effects of strychnine poison.

However, under cross-examination by Mr Chandos Leigh, Professor Taylor was willing to entertain the contentious possibility that whilst the child was a probable victim of strychnine, Elizabeth Vamplew may have been a victim of biology. According to Professor Taylor, any girl of the prisoner's age suffering from obstructed menstruation would be likely to suffer 'peculiar effects'. What he meant by 'peculiar effects' was that she might become 'wayward' and subject to 'a strange state of mind under which acts amounting to crime might be committed'. In short, he accepted, at least hypothetically, that Elizabeth Vamplew may not have been completely rational at the time of the administration of poison to Kate Mary Taylor and was therefore not entirely responsible for her actions.

The coverage of the witness statements had added interesting material not heard from the reports on the three inquests and on the hearing in front of the magistrates. However, it was the very lengthy report of the summing up of the case for the Defence by Mr Chandos Leigh which probably engaged the reader of the *Lincolnshire Chronicle* as much as the uncomfortable sensational details heard from the witness stand.

His opening gambit, predictably, was to highlight the prisoner at the bar being a 'poor child', whom he had been called upon to defend 'at the last moment'. The intention to create an object of pity from the sight of a painfully thin thirteen-year old, barely four feet eight inches tall, seated in front of the jury, would not have been difficult.

Equally predictable was his self-ingratiation with the jury, whom he believed would reach a verdict based upon the evidence alone, rather than upon any prejudicial rumours which they may have heard outside the courtroom. He was absolutely confident that the jury would 'look at the case in all its bearings and temper justice with mercy'.

The deferential niceties completed, Mr Chandos Leigh switched to the more prosaic line of text book exposition relating to the cause of death, the agent of that cause and, finally, whether the act causing death was carried out feloniously with malice aforethought.

As Elizabeth Vamplew had confessed to the killing of Kate Mary Taylor, it was clear that the Counsel for the Defence had little choice other than to accept that she would be found Guilty, and that he would probably have to argue for leniency on the grounds of any extenuating circumstances which might modify the concept of 'malice aforethought'.

Pragmatic good sense told the Defence Counsel that it would be pointless to argue against the obvious: the evidence presented 'by the eminent medical witness' was apparently incontrovertible - Kate Mary Taylor had died from strychnine poison.

The second question, as to whether the poison had been administered by the prisoner at the bar, was less clear cut. Apart from her own confessions, there was little evidence to bring a conviction, the Learned Counsel insisted. He conceded that it was the jury who must decide upon how much weight to attach to those confessions; but at the same time, it should bear in mind the possibility that 'in the excitement of the moment' words may have been said for reasons which were totally disconnected from the death of the child.

In a spirit of disingenuous gallantry, Mr Chandos Leigh insisted that he would not have a single word said against Mrs and Mrs Taylor. However, he felt obliged to express his unease at 'the habit of cross-questioning' which had produced the confessions of the prisoner. It was a key issue for the jury to consider and decide as to whether the supposed confessions of the prisoner 'were of such a nature as could be uttered by one who actually administered the poison'. In the version of this section of the Defence Counsel's speech published in *The Sun* newspaper, Mr Chandos Leigh appeared to have been a little more forthright in his comments upon the various interrogations of Elizabeth Vamplew. In his view, her so-called confessions had been made 'under the influence of terror' and that she had been subjected to questions 'which no magistrate, not even his Lordship, had authority to put'.

In a spirit of disingenuous generosity, he continued his defence of Elizabeth Vamplew by allowing the possibility that the poison had been administered out of malice and with forethought, but for that possibility to be accepted by the jury, the Counsel for the Prosecution would have had to have demonstrated a motive. In the opinion of Mr Chandos Leigh, 'no assignable cause for the action had been adduced' by the Learned Counsel. Having said that, he mockingly admitted that there had been 'a semblance' of a motive which had been 'slightly alluded to' in that it was reported that the prisoner had said that 'she was tired of hugging the little thing about'. This shred of evidence against the accused, he suggested, was completely contradicted by Mrs Taylor herself, who had distinctly said that the girl 'had not the care of that child'. In actual fact, if the newspaper report was correct, what Mrs Taylor had said under cross-examination was that it had been the prisoner's duty 'to attend to the other children.'

In unpromising circumstances, Mr Chandos Leigh was trying to meticulously build a case for the Defence out of flimsy shreds and patches. His continuation, however, was perhaps decisive in at least disrupting a straightforward narrative of a calculated act of unspeakable malice. Reminding the jury of the age of Elizabeth Vamplew, he tentatively suggested the possibility that she was unaware of the deadly nature of *Battle's Vermin Killer*, mistakenly thinking that it was just a means of inducing sleep. Given the deposition of Mary Wright in which she claimed to have alerted Elizabeth Vamplew to the dangers of the packet of poison which she had sold to her, it did not seem a very promising line of defence. However, the Learned Counsel further reminded the jury that they had earlier heard Mrs Taylor say that she had sent for an old woman when her daughter was very ill, who had said that 'some sleepy stuff' had been given to the child. Whilst the suggestion was not entirely convincing, it at least invited the jury to consider the concept of accidental poisoning: in a society where opiate-based cordials were often used in the home and in the field to subdue a fretful baby it would have had some credibility. If the child had been accidently poisoned it was, he admitted, an act of criminal negligence, but one which supported his supposition that the intention had been to 'temporarily quiet the child'.

Perhaps in an attempt to firm up his defence of the young girl, Mr Chandos Leigh moved away from the subjective interpretations of words and actions to the more secure ground of legal ruling.

The law set down that any child under the age of seven years old was not responsible for its actions. As far as a child between the age of seven and fourteen was concerned, there was flexibility in the justice system in that the jury had the right to determine whether or not any child charged with an offence had reached 'such a point of intelligence as to be capable of committing a crime with malice aforethought'.

In an attempt to shape the jury's thinking on the issue, the Learned Counsel also alluded to the comment made by Professor Swaine Taylor concerning the subject of obstructed menstruation and its possible impact on adolescent behaviour. Interestingly, Mr Chandos Leigh's description of the condition, as reported by the newspaper, was a good deal more coy and was watered down by qualifying phrases concerning its absolute validity as credible evidence. He reminded the jury of the probability that Elizabeth Vamplew, at her age, was 'under the influence of a peculiar disease which rendered her, *to an extent*, irresponsible *at times* for acts *similar* to the one with which she was charged'. If this was the case, he implored the jury to consider whether they were perfectly satisfied that the expressions which the prisoner had used in confessing to the crime proved her guilt absolutely.

He concluded his address by maintaining that a verdict of criminal negligence would serve the ends of justice. The crime of Elizabeth Vamplew would be atoned for by 'a period of wholesome discipline' which would 'restore her to the path she had forsaken', and in due course, she might become 'a good and useful member of society'.

As an optimistic statement of the mid-Victorian belief in the wholesome influence of a lengthy stay in prison on criminal behaviour, it was admirable; as a prediction of a better future for the thirteen year old girl from Grimoldby, it was woefully inaccurate.

After having heard the case for the Defence, Chief Baron Pollock congratulated Mr Chandos Leigh on his performance: had the Learned Counsel received instructions weeks ago he could not have put the case more clearly. It was a familiar judicial indulgence, but in this case it was as true as it was probably well meant: he had constructed a coherent case which made best use of the available opportunities to undermine an absolute verdict of Guilty, without losing sight of the fact that a baby had lost its life in dreadful circumstances.

It was also clear from His Lordship's summary that he was uneasy about the possibility of a girl of thirteen being found Guilty of murder and of him having to don the black cap, no matter how strong a recommendation for mercy might be from the jury.

After rehearsing the facts of the case, he took the opportunity to remind the jury of the difference between manslaughter and murder. More specifically, he repeated the legal position noted by Mr Chandos Leigh of a jury having the power to determine whether a prisoner charged with a serious crime 'had arrived at that maturity of knowledge as to be capable, in a legal sense, of committing the grave offence'. The Chief Baron's description of the jury's legal entitlement to make such a judgement as 'very humane and just', made it clear where his sympathies lay.

The account of this section of the judge's summing up by the *Lincolnshire Chronicle* might be supplemented by that found in *The Sun*, which includes to a preamble apparently omitted by the

Lincoln newspaper. Before summing up the evidence, the he had recalled a case of over sixty years ago when a jury had found a prisoner Guilty of wilful murder, but then had immediately recommended a reprieve. The Chief Baron had been struck by the 'strange inconsistency' of a prisoner being rightfully convicted of wilful murder being deemed to deserve an immediate remission from the death sentence. In the context of the trial of Elizabeth Vamplew, rather than being a random caveat, it seemed an undisguised directing of the jury towards a verdict of Not Guilty of wilful murder.

The final words to the jury reported in the *Lincolnshire Chronicle* were a formal objective summary of the legal position, but with a clear cautionary edge to them. Before convicting the child, (as opposed to the prisoner), the jury must 'without doubt be satisfied that there was an adequate motive' and that 'she fully knew what she was doing'; and finally, they must be clear that she was 'of full maturity of intelligence and was conscious of the enormity of the act'.

On the crucial issue of the need for certainty, the Chief Baron could not have been more explicit.

It may have surprised him six years later, had he been able to access a copy of the *Trinidad Chronicle* of 15th September, 1868, that his words were being quoted in the Supreme Criminal Court of the island by Mr James Fitzjames Stephen, when defending a certain Mr Kallowah, who was accused of stabbing a woman to death. In the case of Regina v Vamplew, said Mr Stephens, Chief Baron Pollock had insisted upon the key concept of the accused being fully conscious of the fatal effect of their action and that any lack of certainty on this issue precluded a verdict of wilful murder. Unfortunately for Mr Stephen, the Vamplew case, quite rightly, was not considered relevant by the judge and that the Learned Counsel had 'laid down the wrong law'; unfortunately for Mr Kallowah, the jury agreed and he was sentenced to death.

The jury took just five minutes to decide that Elizabeth Vamplew was guilty of manslaughter: the sentence was deferred, but later confirmed as twelve years penal servitude.

The *Lincolnshire Chronicle* ended its report by noting that many people present in court were 'considerably affected by the exceedingly juvenile appearance of the prisoner'. In its lack of the usual journalistic hyperbole and sensationalism, the quietly understated description of thirteen year old Elizabeth Vamplew sitting in the dock and seldomly raising her eyes during the proceedings, was probably an accurate one.

The *Stamford Mercury*, which had also been following the case, reported on the trial and in most respects duplicated that of the *Lincolnshire*

Chronicle. However, there were some occasional interesting departures from the Lincoln newspaper's version of events in terms of both content, emphasis and tone.

The opening paragraph of the report created a very different image of Elizabeth Vamplew which immediately orientated the reader's reception of the subsequent narrative of the trial. The prisoner in the dock was 'a little girl of about 13 years of age' - that was about as sympathetic as it got; her 'gloomy expression of countenance' indicated 'a vindictive disposition', according to the reporter.

The intellectually bankrupt excursion into the medieval pseudo-science of Physiognomy in order to explain the anxieties of a child trapped in a bewildering adult world of weird words, fancy wigs and polished wood, was not encouraging. Even more discouraging was the description of the opening of the formal procedures in which Elizabeth Vamplew pleaded Guilty to the charge of murder. The conclusion of the reporter was that she did not know the meaning or the consequences of her plea. That she did not understand the legal consequences was probably true, but the suggestion that she did not understand the concept of an admission of guilt was questionable.

If the assertion that Elizabeth Vamplew was completely baffled by what she was being asked is true, what was reported next bordered on the downright bizarre. According to the *Stamford Mercury*, in order to get her to change her mind, the prisoner was asked the very same question again, using the exact terms of reference that she had allegedly not understood in the first place.

The report in the *Lincolnshire Chronicle* passed over the Counsel for the Prosecution's opening speech with only a brief reference to it and without going into specifics; the *Stamford Mercury*, on the other hand, gave a precise, point by point, account of the key arguments. Consequently, the depositions of the witnesses were less detailed than in the *Lincolnshire Chronicle*.

The exception to this was the evidence related by and to Mary Taylor, the mother of the poisoned infant, which foregrounded her part in the domestic tragedy.

In his opening speech, Mr Sargeaunt told the court that it was Mary Taylor who had given Elizabeth Vamplew permission to go to the school feast at Grimoldby on the 10th July and that during that time she nursed her infant daughter all day and the child was perfectly well in her care. Edwin Taylor, in his deposition, confirmed what the Learned Counsel had said about this wife, and re-iterated that on seeing 'the suffering of the child', she had fainted.

In her deposition, Mrs Taylor, 'attired in deep

mourning', insisted that she had never asked the prisoner to buy mouse poison; and further, in a declaration more damning than that reported in the *Lincolnshire Chronicle*, 'She *always* suspected her of being a very deceitful girl'.

Whilst the depositions of all of the witnesses were noted, there was no record of any of the cross-examinations, by either the Counsel for the Prosecution or the Defence.

The final speech by Edward Chandos Leigh on behalf of the prisoner was reported, although not in the kind of detail found in the *Lincolnshire Chronicle*. Arguments put forward by Mr Chandos Leigh were noted in a very superficial manner or in slightly different words.

The most interesting part of this version of the speech, was the section relating to the suggestion by Professor Swaine Taylor that issues relating to adolescent menstruation might be considered as a factor in the case. If the *Lincolnshire Chronicle*'s version of the words of the Counsel for the Defence was quite obviously trying to convey a sanitised account of the medical man's evidence for public consumption, that in the *Stamford Mercury* amounted to journalism being held at gun point by Mrs Grundy. On account of 'certain peculiar conditions of the system, females were possessed with strange delusions, which rendered them unaccountable beings'. Mr Chandos

Leigh, it was reported, had endeavoured 'to draw an inference that the prisoner might have been suffering under a similar disease'.

It was perhaps with some relief that the reporter was able to inform his readers that no precise evidence was presented to the court to support such an indelicate possibility.

After summarising the recapitulation of the evidence by Chief Baron Pollock, the newspaper reported that the jury reached a verdict of manslaughter, but only after 'a prolonged deliberation', which was a something of a contrast to the five minutes claimed by the *Lincolnshire Chronicle*.

On being sentenced at the Assizes, Elizabeth Vamplew was returned to Lincoln Castle prison where she remained until the 1st September, when she was removed to Millbank in Surrey, along with the prisoners William Elwood, William Porter and John Fell. The Prison Governor had written a letter requesting her transfer on 11th August, but the process seems to have been delayed by the need for the Prison Surgeon to treat her for stomach pains and also for a non-infectious rash on her chest.

After seven months and sixteen days, she was removed from the unhealthy dampness of Millbank to Parkhurst prison on the Isle of Wight; after thirty-eight months and sixteen days, she was transferred back to the mainland and spent nine months and twelve days in Brixton prison, before being released on licence by the Home Secretary, on 9th March, 1867.

Throughout her time in prison she appears to have been an exemplary prisoner, her conduct being described as either Good or Very Good, and her educational progress recorded as either Satisfactory or Very Satisfactory.

The *Record of Prison Offences* for Elizabeth Vamplew shows that she was never 'awarded' any additional punishments for breaches of the rules.

Her prison trades, consisting of knitting and needlework, earned her an average monthly wage of just over £7 during her time at Parkhurst and Brixton prisons, before returning home to Grimoldby.

Aftermath

The trial and conviction of Elizabeth Vamplew was reported widely throughout the United Kingdom in various truncated and redacted versions, with the young girl being particularly demonised by Scottish newspapers.

One unexpected story which emerged from some of these reports was the belief that Elizabeth Vamplew had killed other infants. In some versions, such as the *Worcester Chronicle* of 6th August, the report was circumspect, only suggesting that the facts of the case 'tend to fix the death of two other infants on the prisoner'; whilst other publications, such as the *Sheffield Independent* of 4th August and the *Durham County Advertiser* of 8th August, were less compromising, and described the possibility of multiple murders as 'a strong belief'.

The Hereford Times and General Advertiser of 16th August was especially robust in its presentation of Elizabeth Vamplew as a mass murderer in a lurid article titled, 'Murders and Attempts to Murder'. The youthful poisoner had been convicted of one murder, but was almost certainly guilty of several, according to the newspaper. Rehashing the alleged words of Chief Baron Pollock, the article claimed that she knew more about the death of two other infants than she had let on. In conclusion, she was 'a person exceedingly dangerous to those with whom she might be associated' and was prone 'under the influence of some unknown but horrible nature, to this dreadful form of crime'.

The unrestrained and outraged hyperbole, as well as the surrounding context which told of gruesome and distressing depravity from Doncaster to Isleworth in order to prove the newspaper's claim that 'murders are rife just now', may have tested the credulity of the reader to the limit.

It was not unusual for newspapers to invent sensational stories after a murder trial which heaped further ignominy on the accused: Eliza Joyce, for example, convicted in Lincoln of killing her own children with laudanum in 1844, supposedly murdered a young lover as well as her own father, according to one mischievous newspaper account. However, the claim that Elizabeth Vamplew probably killed at least two other infants was not entirely without foundation and was given both credence and respectability by Professor Swaine Taylor three years later.

During the trial, it was recollected by Edwin Taylor that Elizabeth Vamplew had mentioned in passing that her infant sister and the baby of Mrs Bromby had died in similar circumstances to Kate Mary Taylor. Moreover, she commented, as a matter of fact, that the child of Mrs Bromby had taken an hour and a quarter to die. Whilst it was hardly indisputable evidence that Elizabeth Vamplew had anything to do with the death of the two infants, it may well have produced a sense of uneasiness in court.

That Swaine Taylor had chosen to draw attention to the Vamplew case is not surprising, as at the end of the trial the foreman of the jury had handed a piece of paper to Chief Baron Pollock which highlighted the dangers of the indiscriminate sale of the poison such as that sold to Elizabeth Vamplew. In the words of the *Lincolnshire Chronicle*, on receiving the piece of paper, the judge had said that 'the Grand Jury had made a very proper representation, and he would take care that it was forwarded to the Secretary for the Home Department'. He added that he had been astonished that a woman should have 'unlimited power of disposing of an article calculated to spread death and destruction around the community': it was a statement which captured the blinkered mindset of a mid-Victorian judge, as much as a sense of the urgent need for government regulation.

In the course of arguing for greater regulation

in *The Pharmaceutical Journal and Transactions*, Professor Taylor also drew attention to the death of two other infants from the administration of *Battle's Vermin Killer*. According to the expert toxicologist, Elizabeth Vamplew had acted as a nurse to infants in families other than the Taylors, and that on previous occasions, the infants entrusted in her care had died suddenly of convulsions and, in addition, it was believed that those convulsions were a result of the administration of *Battle's Vermin Killer*.

With the publication of Professor Swaine Taylor's paper, Elizabeth Vamplew became a footnote in the history of judicial toxicology. She was soon, however, to become a footnote in the annals of English prison history.

Mr Chandos Leigh, in his closing remarks for the Defence, had expressed the solemn hope that a substantial prison term would improve the moral character of Elizabeth Vamplew and, in due course, transform her into a good and useful member of society. The optimism of his predicted reclamation of the young girl from criminality was never fully tested, despite her apparently unblemished prison record.

Elizabeth Vamplew was released from Brixton prison on licence having served less than half of her twelve year sentence. The conditions of the licence, signed by Spencer Herbert Walpole a couple of months before his resignation as Home Secretary, were clear and unequivocal: any breach would lead her inexorably back to prison for seven years and four months.

It hardly mattered.

Elizabeth Vamplew was granted a 'licence to be at large' based 'on medical grounds', rather than for reasons of good behaviour: she died just over nine months later, aged eighteen years.

Her death, like her life, was somewhat strange and enigmatic. The *Grimoldby Burial Register* records the interment of Elizabeth Vamplew on the 18th December, 1869, just eleven days after that of her mother, Maria Vamplew, aged forty-eight.

It was a curiously sombre joining together of the two women, recorded respectively as number 355 and 356 in the burial register, after the apparent dissension in the courtroom seven years earlier.

Postscript

The identity of Elizabeth Vamplew after she was indicted for the murder of Kate Mary Taylor was defined by court rooms and newspapers: in both contexts, she was primarily a self-confessed child murderer and therefore a judicial problem in need of a judicial solution. The fundamental requirements of that solution were that they addressed the needs of the grieving parents and, at the same time, the demands of the law: both involved redress and punishment. The solution of twelve years of penal servitude seemed to satisfy both parties: Elizabeth Vamplew was punished for administering poison to an infant, Elizabeth Vamplew was removed from respectable society and Elizabeth Vamplew was deprived of her freedom for a very long time.

Once absorbed into the prison system, the identity of Elizabeth Vamplew acquired additional attributes. In the Assize Calendar she had been numbered

949, but once convicted of manslaughter, she was re-numbered 194, moving between the prisons of Lincoln, Millbank, Parkhurst and Brixton. As well as the details of her trial and incarceration, Elizabeth Vamplew's identity was also defined in the spare, bureaucratic inventory written by James Foster, the Governor of Lincoln Castle, on the eve of her transfer to Millbank. Prisoner 194 had a fair complexion, light brown hair, grey eyes, was four foot eight inches tall and thin. Her defining characteristics were two deformed front teeth on the upper jaw and a mole on her left breast.

That Elizabeth Vamplew was a mere child was acknowledged in court and in the media, although with little sense of any deep understanding of the human implications of what was happening to a girl of thirteen. The exchanges in court between the Learned Counsels drew attention to the fact of her age, but primarily in terms of the legal issues of intent and moral responsibility, enabling the jury to avoid the possibility of the death penalty with a clear conscience. Some newspaper reporters observed the confusions of a child caught up the judicial process, yet at the same time only existing on its margins, both socially and linguistically. But such an image was more a contrived pathos to satisfy the needs of a sensationalist narrative than a genuine concern for the fate of a daughter of an obscure Grimoldby farm labourer, trying to make sense of a world which was not her own.

During the course of the trial, the identity of Elizabeth Vamplew was not that of an isolated scrawny child who had asked for a penny dolly at the village shop, but rather of the scheming purchaser of strychnine in a three-penny packet, who was intent on murder.

The depositions of the key witnesses, in passing, provided the court with the briefest of snapshots of Elizabeth Vamplew before her arrest and indictment, which amounted to little more than supplementary confirmations of her criminal identity. Her employer, Mary Taylor, had always thought her to be a deceitful young girl and therefore not to be trusted - a perception reinforced by Edwin Taylor's pressing questions about the mystery contents of a bottle and the hidden contents of her box. Betsy Clarke's recollections defined her as lacking any kind of empathy with human misfortune when she was told of the agonised death of an infant which she had probably just poisoned, yet having the supreme self-confidence to dismiss the competence of a coroner's jury to uncover the truth.

To the moral imperfection of deceitfulness, both Edwin Taylor and his father-in-law added the criminal imperfection of social deviancy, when they recalled the chilling detachment of Elizabeth

Vamplew's recollections of infant poisonings in the area, including that of her own sister.

The trial required no discussion of motive as the accused had freely admitted to killing Kate Mary Taylor, although according to William Mitchell, based upon his conversation with her, Elizabeth Vamplew had been merely fed up with carrying the child around. It was a slightly implausible claim, although not unique in nineteenth century trials of domestic servants, some of who saw the children in their care as an annoying additional chore on top of many.

More pressing was a rational explanation for such an incomprehensible act of cruelty by a child towards an infant. This was left to Edward Chandos Leigh, who tentatively suggested a possible lack of awareness of the destructive power of certain powders, and to Alfred Swaine Taylor, who concurred, at least hypothetically, that blocked menstruation might result in abnormal patterns of behaviour.

The more robust explanation of the *Hereford Times and General Advertiser*, that the thirteen year old girl was influenced by an aberrant nature was probably more acceptable to the 'startled and shocked reader' than the subtleties of any Defence Counsel or the uncertainties of a Professor of Medical Jurisprudence, no matter how distinguished.

Given the absence of reliable detailed information about Elizabeth Vamplew, it is difficult to explain her destructive actions with any confidence, without resorting to speculation.

However, what few fragments of fact we do possess perhaps prompts questions which a Victorian court would not have entertained as admissible or even relevant to an understanding of the crime.

Elizabeth Vamplew was from an impoverished background in the small agricultural community of Grimoldby, about five miles east of Louth. In the 1861 Census, she was living with her father John Vamplew, an agricultural labourer, and his wife Maria, along with her two sisters, Susan (aged ten), Anna (aged seven) and her brother Edwin, (aged three). The baby of the family, Charlotte, was buried on Census day, aged around eight months. Both John and Maria Vamplew were born in Grimoldby, as were all the children of the marriage: their existence seemed to be circumscribed and defined entirely by the narrow confines of Grimoldby.

Other members of the family lived close by: Susannah Vamplew, aged seventy-five and recorded as a grocer's widow and a pauper, lived next door, along with Henry Vamplew, her son, aged thirty-one, who was a farm servant, whilst two doors away lived Philip Bratby and his family, who was the brother of Maria Vamplew.

Mid-century life in Grimoldby seems to have been stolid, steady and unruffled until around 1865 when the area was panicked by an outbreak of rinderpest, a highly infectious viral disease which destroyed livestock and livelihoods.

The ethos of the village was defined mainly by the moral improvement agenda of the Wesleyans, the Primitive Methodists and Free Methodists: all three had established chapels in the village by 1855. One of the probable highlights of the social life of Grimoldby was the celebration of the anniversary of the Free Methodist Sunday School, which was clearly important enough and exciting enough for a thirteen year old girl to attend. In July 1863, the festivities included a seaside outing to Mablethorpe for the children, enabled by Mr Foster of Cockerington, which the *Louth and North Lincolnshire Advertiser* described as 'an unrestrained romp'. At this point in time, Elizabeth Vamplew was neither unrestrained nor enjoying a playful romp on the beach, having been recently transferred to Parkhurst prison on the Isle of Wight from Millbank.

For some time, there had been a serious concern in the area over a lack of adequate provision for the education of the children of the village, and also nearby Manby. By March, 1866, thanks to the efforts and generosity of the Reverend W T Towers, rector of Grimoldby, and the Reverend J D Waite, rector of Manby, plus the principal property owners of the area, a 'handsome and commodious building' was established. Nominally, it was a Church of England school, but was open to all Christian denominations.

Up to that point, local children had been given only a rudimentary education in a Grimoldby cottage, bequeathed in 1780 by the Reverend Francis Burton for the use of the poor. In 1856, William White noted the existence of the cottage and the fact that it was currently occupied by paupers; he also noted that the overseers of the parish paid a yearly fee of five pounds to a schoolmaster, specifically for teaching the children of the poor.

The prison authorities assessed the reading and writing capabilities of Elizabeth Vamplew as 'imperfect', a vague and flexible word which at best meant that they were not very good. However, she may have had a very basic proficiency, acquired at the cottage house in the 1850s, before entering service in May, 1862, at the house of Mr and Mrs Taylor.

The employment history of Elizabeth Vamplew before the traditional hiring date of the 1st May in 1862 is both vague and in a sense contentious.

Before working for the Taylors, she had been employed for only five weeks in the service of Mary Wright, the village shop keeper. What she did and when, as well as why she left the service of Mrs Wright, is unknown: it may be that the arrangement was a purely casual one agreed on a temporary basis.

The more pressing questions relate to whether

Elizabeth Vamplew was helping out her mother at home by looking after her baby sister, Charlotte, around the time of her premature death in April 1861; and also, whether or not she was employed by William and Mary Bromby in any capacity which would have given her access to their son.

The answers are more than of academic interest in that Professor Swaine Taylor was quite insistent that two infants died in suspicious circumstances and that Elizabeth Vamplew was indisputably implicated: 'It turned out upon inquiry that this child had acted as nurse to infants in other families; and on two previous occasions, *the infants entrusted to her care* had also died suddenly in convulsions, as it is believed from the administration of this deadly poison!' In an article written by an expert in medical jurisprudence and published in an established medical journal, what was reported in the newspapers as an unsubstantiated allegation was now likely to secure the status of accepted fact.

In the light of such retrospective certainty, it seems all the more remarkable that Mr and Mrs Taylor should have entrusted the care of their infant daughter to a young girl associated, even if only by suspicious circumstances and tenuous local gossip, with the sudden death of two infants in the area.

The confident assertion of Swaine Taylor conveniently supported his broad theme of the appalling dangers of vermin killers in the wrong hands and, at the same time, created the identity of Elizabeth Vamplew as a monstrous multiple murderer of infants. It was an identity to some extent built upon the behaviours and words deposed in court by several witnesses, which suggested a disquieting lack of concern about the death of Kate Mary Taylor by the accused.

What is certain is that the possible re-invention of Elizabeth Vamplew by Swaine Taylor as a fearful monster, who murdered tiny children without compunction with strychnine, left little space for the equally plausible identity of a disturbed and bewildered child, incapable of processing the true horror of her actions.

It is perhaps significant that in every media account of what took place in Alvingham, no matter how sympathetic, her identity was pared down to that of Elizabeth Vamplew, the remorseless poisoner.

It seems that she was never allowed to be the alternative oversimplification of Lizzie Vamplew, aged thirteen, a girl who still dandled and patted penny dolls.

Key Players in the Life of Elizabeth Vamplew

ANDERSON, Honourable Charles Henry John. Served on the Grand Jury at the trial of Elizabeth Vamplew. Resident of Lea Hall, near Gainsborough.

BACON, Henry Hickman. Served on the Grand Jury at the trial of Elizabeth Vamplew. Resident of Thonock Hall, Gainsborough.

BEAUCLERK, Lord Frederick Charles Peter. On the Bench of Louth Magistrate's Court. Resident of The Hall, Little Grimsby.

BROMBY, Mary. Mother of William Ingleby Bromby. Resident of Manby Hall.

BROMBY, William Ingleby. Possible murder victim of Elizabeth Vamplew. Resident of Manby Hall.

CAVE, Lewis. Counsel for the Prosecution at the trial of Elizabeth Vamplew, at the Lincoln Assizes.

CHAPLIN, Colonel Thomas. Served on the Grand Jury at the trial of Elizabeth Vamplew.

CHOLMELEY, Sir Montague John. MP for North Lincolnshire. Served on the Grand Jury at the trial of Elizabeth Vamplew. Resident of Easton Hall.

CLARKE, Betsy. Domestic servant employed by Edwin Taylor. Gave evidence at the inquest into the death Kate Mary Taylor, as well as at the magistrates' court in Louth, and at the trial of Elizabeth Vamplew at the Lincoln Assizes. Resident of Alvingham.

CORBETT, Thomas George. Served on the Grand Jury at the trial of Elizabeth Vamplew. Resident of Elsham Hall.

ELLISON, Richard. Banker. Served on the Grand Jury at the trial of Elizabeth Vamplew. Resident of Sudbrooke Holme.

FOSTER, James: Governor of Lincoln Castle.

FFYTCHE, John Lewis. Served on the Grand Jury at the trial of Elizabeth Vamplew. Resident of Thorpe Hall, South Elkington.

HAMILTON, Sir Robert North Collie Hamilton. Served on the Grand Jury at the trial of Elizabeth Vamplew. Resident of Avon Cliffe, Stratford-upon-Avon, Warwickshire.

HENEAGE, George Fieschi. Served on the Grand Jury at the trial of Elizabeth Vamplew. Resident of Hainton Hall.

HUTTON, William. Served on the Grand Jury at the trial of Elizabeth Vamplew.

JARVIS, George Knowles. Served on the Grand Jury at the trial of Elizabeth Vamplew. Resident of Doddington Hall.

LEIGH, Honourable Edward Chandos. Counsel for the Defence at the trial of Elizabeth Vamplew at the Lincoln Assizes. Resident of Stoneleigh Abbey, Warwickshire.

MASSINGBERD-MUNDY, Charles. Served on the Grand Jury at the trial of Elizabeth Vamplew. Resident of Ormsby Hall.

MELVILLE, Honourable Alexander Leslie. Banker. Served on the Grand Jury at the trial of Elizabeth Vamplew. Resident of Branston Hall.

MITCHELL, William. Farmer. Gave evidence at the inquest into the death Kate Mary Taylor, his granddaughter, and at the trial of Elizabeth Vamplew at the Lincoln Assizes.

MOORE, Charles Thomas James. Served on the Grand Jury at the trial of Elizabeth Vamplew. Resident of Frampton Hall.

NEVILLE, George. Served on the Grand Jury at the trial of Elizabeth Vamplew. Resident of Stubton Hall.

PACKE, George Hussey. Served on the Grand Jury at the trial of Elizabeth Vamplew. Resident of Caythorpe Hall.

PARKER, William. Served on the Grand Jury at the trial of Elizabeth Vamplew. Resident of Westgate, Louth.

PEACOCK, Reverend Wilkinson Affleck. Served on the Grand Jury at the trial of Elizabeth Vamplew. Resident of Rectory House, Ulceby.

POLLOCK, Chief Baron Frederick. Judge at the trial of Elizabeth Vamplew at the Lincoln Assizes.

PYE, H. Solicitor. On the Bench at the Magistrates' Court, Louth. Resident of Westgate, Louth.

REEVE, John. Served on the Grand Jury at the trial of Elizabeth Vamplew. Resident of Leadenham House.

RICHTER, Reverend Henry William. Chaplain of Lincoln Castle Prison and Rector of St Paul in the Bail, Lincoln. Resident of 23 Minster Yard, Lincoln.

ROBERTS, Inspector William. Louth policeman. Arrested and charged Elizabeth Vamplew. Gave evidence at the inquest into the death Kate Mary Taylor and at the trial of Elizabeth Vamplew at the Lincoln Assizes.

SARGEAUNT, John B. Counsel for the Prosecution at the trial of Elizabeth Vamplew, at the Lincoln Assizes.

SHARPLEY, Dr Thomas. Presiding coroner at the inquest into the death of Kate Mary Taylor. Resident of Eastgate, Louth.

SMYTH, Reverend William. On the Bench of the Magistrates' Court, Louth. Resident of Thorpe Hall, South Elkington.

SMYTH, William Henry. Chairman of the Magistrates' Bench at Louth and served on the Grand Jury at the trial of Elizabeth Vamplew. Resident of Thorpe Hall, South Elkington.

TAYLOR, Professor Alfred Swaine. Professor of Medical Jurisprudence at Guy's Hospital, London. Gave evidence at the resumed inquest into the death Kate Mary Taylor and at the trial of Elizabeth Vamplew at the Lincoln Assizes.

TAYLOR, Kate Mary. Daughter of Edwin and Mary Taylor. Resident of Alvingham.

TAYLOR, Edwin. Farmer. Gave evidence at the inquest into the death Kate Mary Taylor, his daughter, as well as at the magistrates' court in Louth and at the trial of Elizabeth Vamplew at the Lincoln Assizes. Resident of Alvingham.

TAYLOR, Mary. Wife of Edwin Taylor. Gave evidence at the inquest into the death Kate Mary Taylor, her daughter, as well as at the magistrates' court in Louth and at the trial of Elizabeth Vamplew at the Lincoln Assizes. Resident of Alvingham.

TROLLOPE, Right Honourable Sir John. Served on the Grand Jury at the trial of Elizabeth Vamplew. Resident of Casewick House, near Uffington.

VAMPLEW, Charlotte. Sister of Elizabeth Vamplew.

Possible murder victim of Elizabeth Vamplew. Resident of Grimoldby.

VAMPLEW, Maria. Mother of Elizabeth Vamplew. Gave evidence at the inquest into the death Kate Mary Taylor, at the magistrates' court in Louth and at the Lincoln Assizes. Resident of Grimoldby.

WALPOLE, Honourable Spencer Herbert. Home Secretary. Signed Conditional Licence for release of Elizabeth Vamplew from Brixton prison.

WELBY, William Earle. Served on the Grand Jury at the trial of Elizabeth Vamplew. Resident of Denton Hall.

WILLSON, Anthony. Served on the Grand Jury at the trial of Elizabeth Vamplew. Resident of Rauceby Hall.

WRIGHT, Mary. Wife of John Wright, shopkeeper. Gave evidence at the inquest into the death Kate Mary Taylor, at the magistrates' court in Louth and at the trial of Elizabeth Vamplew at the Lincoln Assizes. Resident of Grimoldby.

WROE, John B. Surgeon. Gave evidence at the inquest into the death Kate Mary Taylor and at the trial of Elizabeth Vamplew at the Lincoln Assizes. Resident of 140 Eastgate, Louth.

BIBLIOGRAPHY

Chapter One

Archive sources
Lincolnshire Archives, Lincoln
Commonplace book belonging to Mary Thorald, 1812
Ref: THOR/12/2/1
Thorald Family, Memorandum Book, 1815-1823
Ref: THOR/12/2/3

Books on Vermin Killing
Anonymous, *The compleat English, French, and High-German vermin-killer. To which is added, directions for curing all sorts of cattle. With some directions for gardiners: being a Companion for all Families shewing A ready way to destroy Adders, Badgers , Birds of all sorts, Bugs, Ducks, Earwigs, Fish, Fleas, flies, Foxes, Frogs, Gnats, Lice, Mice, Otters, Pismires, Polt-Cats,*

Rabits, Rats, Scorpions, Snakes, Snails, Spiders, Toads, Wahts or Miles, Wasps, Weasles, Wolf-fly, Worms in Houses, Gardens et cetera, to which is added Directions for Curing all Sorts of Cattle, With some Directions for Gardiners and the Prozes of Workmen's Labour. Being a Rich Cabinet of Curiosities. (London, *1725*) Wellcome Institute copy: ESTC T473791

Anonymous, *The Vermin-killer: Being a compleat and necessary family-book, shewing a ready way to destroy adders, badgers, birds of all sorts, earwigs, caterpillars, flies, fish, foxes, frogs, gnats, mice, otters, pismires, polecats, rabbets, rats, snakes, scorpions, snails, spiders, toads, wasps, weasles, wants or moles, worms in houses and gardens, bugs, lice, fleas, &c. Also several excellent receipts for the cure of most disorders. And some useful directions for gardening and husbandry; and likewise for travellers in regard to the management of a horse on a journey, &c. With many curious secrets in art and nature,* (Printed and sold by W. Owen, at Homer's Head, near Temple-Bar, London, c.1755) (Wellcome Institute copy: ESTC T200543)

Robert Baldwin, *Multum in parvo; or, everyman His own Vermin-Killer. Containing the most effectual methods of destroying that mischievous little animal the rat; as also the Mouse, Mole, Grasshopper, Ant, Dore, or Blackclock, Worms, Snails, Weasel, Polecat,*

Stoat, and Fox. By a farmer, Who has made it his Study these seven Years. (London, c.1771)
(Wellcome Institute copies: ESTC T41612 and ESTC T208450)

Thomas Simpson, *The Complete Vermin-Killer or Gentleman's and Farmer's Guide for Destroying Water Rats, House Rats, Field Rats, Mice, Moles, Ants or Pissmires, Worms, Snails, Grasshoppers, Crows, Weazels, Polecats, Stoats and Foxes, by Thomas Simpson, Grazier, in the East Riding of Yorkshire*, (Published by John Smith, Bookseller, York, 1772)
(Wellcome Institute copy: ESTC T13164)

Anonymous, *The compleat Vermin-Killer, A Valuable and Useful Companion for Families in Town and Country*, (Fielding & Walker, Pater Noster Row, London, 1777), 2nd edition.
(Wellcome Institute copy: ESTC T66046)

Daniel Holland MD, *The New and Complete Universal Vermin-Killer; being An Infallible Directory for Taking live, destroying, and driving away All Four-footed Creeping, and Winged Vermin, Destructive to Mankind, Dwelling-Houses, Gardens et cetera*, (Printed for Alexander Hogg at the King's Arms, 16 Pater Noster Row, by S Couchman, Throgmorton Street, London, 1802).

Anonymous, *The New and Complete Universal Vermin-Killer; being An Infallible Directory for Taking live, destroying, and driving away All Four-footed Creeping, and Winged Vermin, Destructive to Mankind, Dwelling-Houses, Gardens et cetera*, (Printed by William Darton junior, 58 Holborn Hill, London, 1818).

Anonymous, *The new and complete vermin-killer; being an infallible directory for taking alive, destroying, and driving away vermin, destructive to mankind, dwelling houses, gardens et cetera*, (Dean & Munday, London, 1825)

(Wellcome Institute copy: EPB/P/38536)

Books/Articles

Allen, Alfred Henry, 'Vermin killers containing strychnine', *Pharmaceutical Journal and Transactions*, Third Series, Volume 20, July-December, 1889, pp.296-300

Bartrip, Peter, 'A "pennurth of arsenic for rat poison": the Arsenic Act, 1851, and the prevention of secret poisoning', *Medical History*, 36, 1992, pp.53-69

Macintyre, Ben, *Operation Mincemeat: the True Spy Story that Changed the Course of World War II*, (Bloomsbury: London, 2010), p.51

Taylor, Alfred Swaine, 'Report on Poisoning, and the Dispensing, Vending, and Keeping of Poison', *Pharmaceutical Journal and Transactions*, Second Series, Volume 6, July 1864-June 1865, pp.172-184

Newspapers

Manchester Mercury, 4th November, 1755, p.4
Sussex Advertiser, 17th August, 1761, p.4
Shrewsbury Chronicle, 23rd November, 1776, p.2
Derby Mercury, 19th June, 1778, p.4
Leeds Intelligencer, 19th June, 1781, p.3
Leeds Intelligencer, 17th December, 1792, p.4
Derby Mercury, 16th July, 1793, p.3
Bristol Mercury, 30 August, 1845, p.4
Stamford Mercury, 1st February, 1850, p.3
Lincolnshire Chronicle, 3rd December, 1852, p.8
Bell's Weekly Messenger, 20th December, 1852, p.4
Westmorland Gazette – 14th February 1857, p.6
Derbyshire Advertiser and Journal, 25th September, 1857, p.4
Sheffield Daily Telegraph, 13th November, 1857, p.3
Lincolnshire Chronicle, 12th September, 1862, p.5
Lincolnshire Chronicle, 31st October, 1862, p.7
Grantham Journal, 1st November, 1862, p.2
Lincolnshire Chronicle, 12th December, 1862, p.5
Lincolnshire Chronicle, 19th December, 1862, p.1
Lincolnshire Chronicle, 19th December, 1862, p.8
Boston Guardian, 24th September, 1864, p.2
Cirencester Times and Cotswold Advertiser, 18th June, 1866, p.8
Grantham Journal, 19th March, 1870, p.7
Lincolnshire Chronicle, 8th April, 1870, p.7

Stamford Mercury, 8th April, 1870, p.6
Lincolnshire Chronicle, 20th May, 1870, p.5
Stamford Mercury, 12th May, 1871, p.5
Hull and Eastern Counties Herald, 18th May, 1871, p.7
Lincolnshire Chronicle, 19th May, 1871, p.5
Derbyshire Times and Chesterfield Herald, 20th May, 1871, p.7
Reynolds's Newspaper, 21st May, 1871, p.2
The Illustrated Police News, 27th May, 1871, p.1
Lincolnshire Chronicle, 2nd June, 1871, p.5
Lincolnshire Chronicle, 30th October, 1874, p.7
Lincoln Gazette, 31st October, 1874, p.3
Epworth Bells, Crowle and Isle of Axholme Messenger, 29th March, 1879, p.3
Lincolnshire Chronicle, 11th January, 1881, p.3
Stamford Mercury, 25th February, 1881, p.8
Lincolnshire Chronicle, 8th March, 1881, p.4
Lincolnshire Chronicle, 28th May, 1882, p.7
Grantham Journal, 29th July, 1882, p.4
Grantham Journal, 11th, November, 1882, p.8
Stamford Mercury, 17th November, 1882, p.4
Lincolnshire Chronicle, 9th February, 1883, p.7
Stamford Mercury, 9th February, 1883, p.5
Lincolnshire Chronicle, 22nd June, 1883, p.8
Stamford Mercury, 22nd June, 1883, p.5
Grantham Journal, 23rd June, 1883, p.2
Spalding Guardian, 23rd June, 1883, p.5
Sheffield Daily Telegraph, 12th September, 1889, p.7

Lincolnshire Chronicle, 11th March, 1892, p.7
Sheffield Daily Telegraph, 12th December, 1896, p.11
Horncastle News and South Lindsey Advertiser, 20th February, 1897, p.1
Boston Guardian, 19th December, 1896, p.3
Lincolnshire Echo, 7th December, 1897, p.3
Stamford Mercury, 18th December, 1898, p.5

Chapter Two

Archive sources
Lincolnshire Archives, Lincoln
Prison Journal of James Foster, Governor of Lincoln Castle
Ref: CoC 5/1//5/6: 1860-1868

Prison Journal of Henry W Richter, Chaplain of Lincoln Castle
Ref: CoC 5/1/26: 1861-1866

Prison Journal of Ralph Howett, Surgeon of Lincoln Castle
Ref: CoC 5/1/18

Prison Journal of Gaoler, 1860-1866
Ref: CoC 5/1/4
Prison Journal of Matron, 1860-1878
Ref: CoC 5/1/10

Grimoldby Burial Register, 1813-1967
Ref: Grimoldby PAR/1/8

National Archives, Kew, London
Home Office documents relating to the release of Elizabeth Vamplew under licence
Ref: PCOM 4/32/32
Census Records
1851-1871

Directories
Kelly, E R, *Directory of Lincolnshire with the Port of Hull and Neighbourhood with Map of the County*, various dates
Morris & Co's Commercial Directory and Gazetteer of Lincolnshire, (Hounds Gate, Nottingham, 1863)
White, William, *History, Gazetteer, and the Directory of Lincolnshire and the City and Diocese of Lincoln*, various dates

Newspapers
Louth and North Lincolnshire Advertiser, 12th July, 1862, p.4
Lincolnshire Chronicle, 18th July, 1862, p.7
Stamford Mercury, 18th July, 1862, p.5
Grantham Journal, 19th July, 1862, p.3
Lincolnshire Chronicle, 25th July, 1862, pp.7-8

Louth and North Lincolnshire Advertiser, 26th July, 1862, p.4

The Sun, London, 30th July, 1862, p.8

Leeds Mercury, 31st July, 1862, pp.3-4

Sheffield Independent, 31st July, 1862, p.4

Lincolnshire Chronicle, 1st August, 1862, p.6

Stamford Mercury, 1st August, 1862, p.3

Hull Daily News, 2nd August, 1862, p.5

Louth and North Lincolnshire Advertiser, 2nd August, 1862, p.2

Sheffield Independent, 4th August, 1862, p.3

Shields Daily Gazette, 7th August, 1862, pp.2-3

Southern Reporter, 7th August, 1862, p.4

Coventry Herald and Observer, 8th August, 1862, p.4

Durham County Advertiser, 8th August, 1862, p.3

Louth and North Lincolnshire Advertiser, 9th August, 1862, p.4

Ulverston Mirror and Furness Reflection, 9th August, 1862, pp.3-4

Hereford Times and General Advertiser, 16th August, 1862, p.12

Louth and North Lincolnshire Advertiser, 4th July, 1863, p.4

Louth and North Lincolnshire Advertiser, 16th September, 1865, p.4

Louth and North Lincolnshire Advertiser, 31st March, 1866, p.4

Trinidad Chronicle, 15th September, 1868, p.3

Books/Articles

Gray, Adrian, *Crime and Criminals in Victorian Lincolnshire*, (Paul Watkins: Stamford, 1993), pp.5-6

Taylor, Alfred Swaine, 'Report on Poisoning, and the Dispensing, Vending, and Keeping of Poison', *Pharmaceutical Journal and Transactions*, Second Series, Volume 6, July 1864-June 1865, p.179 and footnote

Watson, Katherine, *Poisoned Lives, English Poisoners and their Victims*, (Hambledon and London, London, 2004), pp.131 and 134 and footnote

General

Anderson, Olive, *Suicide in Victorian and Edwardian England*, (Clarendon Press: Oxford, 1987)

Briggs, Asa, *Victorian Things*, (Batsford Ltd: London, 1988)

Burney, Ian, *Poison, Detection and the Victorian Imagination*, (Manchester University Press: Manchester and New York, 2006)

Moyes, Malcolm, *By Force of Circumstances: the Lefley Case Reopened*, (Matador: Kibworth Beauchamp, 2021)

ibid, Attired in Deepest Mourning – Eliza Joyce, Mary Ann Milner and Priscilla Biggadike, (Matador: Kibworth Beauchamp, 2022) *ibid, Mrs Green's Kettle and other Lincolnshire Acquittals*, (Matador: Kibworth Beauchamp, 2023)

ibid, Reprieved at Lincoln – Lucy Ann Buxton, Emma Wade and Selina Stanhope, (Matador: Kibworth Beauchamp, 2023)

Priestley, Philip, *Victorian Prison Lives*, (Methuen & Co Ltd: London, 1985)

Watson, Katherine, *Poisoned Lives, English Poisoners and their Victims*, (Hambledon and London: London, 2004)

ibid, 'Poisoning Crimes and Forensic Toxicology since the 18th Century', *Academic Forensic Pathology*, Volume 10, Issue 1, March 2020, pp.35-46. Available at https://journals.sagepub.com/doi/full/10.1177/1925362120937923

Whorton, James C, *The Arsenic Century: how Victorian Britain was Poisoned at Home, Work and Play*, (Oxford University Press: Oxford, 2010)

This book is printed on paper from sustainable sources managed under the Forest Stewardship Council (FSC) scheme.

It has been printed in the UK to reduce transportation miles and their impact upon the environment.

For every new title that Matador publishes, we plant a tree to offset CO_2, partnering with the More Trees scheme.

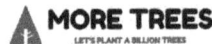

For more about how Matador offsets its environmental impact, see www.troubador.co.uk/about/